THE SKINNY ON DIET SUPPLEMENTS

Fact Vs Fiction

BY
Will Brink

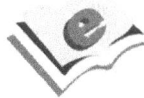

Internet-Publications.net

The Skinny on Diet Supplements: Fact Vs Fiction
Will Brink

Published By
Internet-Publications.net
P.O. Box 1892
Framingham, MA 01701
www.internet-publications.net

Notice of Rights:

Limit of Liability/Disclaimer of Warranty:

Trademarks:

AUTHOR BIO

W ill Brink is a columnist, contributing consultant, and writer for numerous health/fitness, medical, and bodybuilding publications. His articles on nutrition, supplements, weight loss, exercise and medicine can be found in magazines and journals such as "Muscle Insider", "Lets Live," "Muscle Media 2000," "MuscleMag International," "Life Extension," "Muscle & Fitness," "Inside Karate," "Exercise for Men Only," "Oxygen," "The Townsend Letter For Doctors," as well as many international magazines.

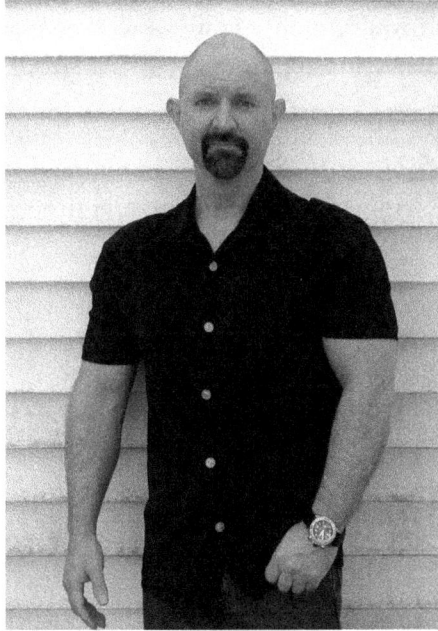

He is the author of the book "Priming The Anabolic Environment: A practical and Scientific Guide to the Art and Science of Building Muscle" and "The Sports Supplement Bible: For Health and Fitness," as well as various chapters in sports nutrition related textbooks. He is also the author of the e-books "Fat Loss Revealed," "Brink's Bodybuilding Revealed."

Will graduated from Harvard University with a concentration in the natural sciences, and is a consultant to supplement companies. He has co-authored several studies relating to sports nutrition and health and published in peer reviewed academic journals.

He has served as an NPC judge and as a Ms. Fitness USA judge. A well-known trainer, Will has helped many top level bodybuilders through all facets of pre-contest and off-season training. He was a Massachusetts Certified Adjunct Trainer at Smith & Wesson Training Academy and has written the book "Practical Applied Stress Training, for Tactical Law Enforcement", named after the class he taught. He has worked with athletes ranging from professional golfers, fitness contestants, police and military personnel.

His articles and interviews can be found on many internet web sites such as: LEF.org, Testosterone.net, NavySeals.com, ThinkMuscle.com, MuscleMonthly.com, as well as many others, including his own site BrinkZone.com.

Will has lectured at trade associations and universities around the United States and has appeared on numerous radio and television programs to examine issues of health and fitness.

Warnings

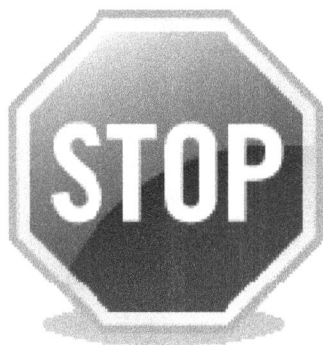

The instructions and advice presented should not be used as a substitute for medical or other personal professional counseling. This book is not intended to give medical advice or replace your doctor.

You should always consult a physician before starting any fat reduction or exercise training program.

A basic metabolic test, thyroid, lipid, cardiovascular and testosterone panel is recommended prior to starting any program in order to detect anything that can prevent you from making the most out of your efforts. Consult your doctor regarding these tests.

You should always speak with your doctor before taking any supplements as they can interfere with any medical therapies or cause problems if you have a medical condition.

CONTENTS AT A GLANCE

TABLE OF CONTENTS

SEPARATING FACT
FROM FICTION

The supplement industry, like all industries, is so full of confusing marketing gimmicks designed to baffle people with BS, people can't make informed decisions as to what to buy or which companies to trust, and that makes it confusing as hell for the average buyer. Never fear, Will Brink is here to explore and explain some of the most common marketing ploys used in supplement ads and product labels that are designed to part you from your money.

The standard fare of slick marketing terms is all too common in the advertising campaigns of some unscrupulous supplement companies, and frankly, they drive me nuts. I've spent 20+ years helping people to make educated, informed decisions regarding the supplements they spend their hard earned money on. What follows is some of the most common marketing terms and what they actually mean to you, the buyer.

Hopefully you can see them for what they really are, and make better decisions about what supplements you buy in the future.

Commonly used marketing terms:

Clinically Proven

Whenever I hear this term I want to call the company up and ask "which clinic and where is it located?" This term means absolutely nothing to the average buyer. What the term is insinuating of course is that the product has been in clinical use for some time and has been found to be effective in a clinical setting, but it's rarely—if ever—true.

Patented

This one of the most powerful of the misleading marketing terms used in the industry. People are under the assumption that a patent means the United States Patent and Trademark Office has evaluated a product and found it to be so effective, it's deserving of a patent. That is simply not the case.

The granting of a patent (and there are several forms of patents, but that's beyond the scope of this book) means the company has an exclusive right to sell the product for the length of the patent, and they have convinced the patent office that idea, or in this case, formula, is original enough to grant a patent.

It does not mean in any way that the product or idea is effective for its intended claim or use, or that it is backed up by legitimate research. One would hope the product was backed up by legitimate research and that's why the patent office granted the patent, but the reality is, this is not the job of the patent office. A patent simply protects a company's legal/financial/intellectual interests.

Translated, there are some really silly patents out there for completely useless and ineffective products. A quick perusal of the patent office web page at http://www.uspto.gov can be fun.

Patents are important and very useful for the company or individual to protect their concept, or product, or what ever the patent is based on from a legal standpoint, so others can't simply take that concept or product and copy it, but it has little to do with efficacy of the product in question. It may be a great product with a patent or it may be a really crappy product with a patent.

Doctor Recommended

Like "clinically proven", I always want to call the company up and ask "which doctor is that and can I have his or her phone number?"

Somehow I know they won't have a doctor for me to talk to. And what type of doctor are they talking about? A medical doctor (MD), or a person with a PhD (also a doctor) in a totally unrelated field? Do I care if a person with a PhD in French History recommends the product? Of course not! Also, does this doctor (or doctors) they have listed in their ad have financial interests in recommending the product or is he doing it out of the goodness of his heart?

The reality is that most MD's have very little knowledge of nutrition or nutritional supplements anyway. Much of the time "Doctor recommended" is a worthless term with no bearing on the effectiveness, quality, or safety of a product, so don't fall for it.

All Natural

I just hate this term! It means nothing at all yet people seem to fall for it virtually every time. Flying is not "natural" to humans, yet we do it all the time. Uranium is natural, but would you want to eat that stuff? Of course not! It's an irrelevant ambiguous term. Ignore it.

Scientifically Formulated

As opposed to what, unscientifically formulated?! Designed by monkeys working on a computer? One would hope the product in question was formulated with some scientific grounding in mind, but this is rarely the case, sad to say. Many products are designed with their marketing power in mind, not their scientific strengths, which leads us to our next term;

Research Proven

If the company has funded legitimate studies at an independent location and the study was published in a peer reviewed journal some place, great! I applaud that company and have for many years lamented about the number of companies that refuse to pay for research to support their own products. The sad fact is, very few companies spend money on real research preferring to spend money on marketing.

If the company has some real research to back up the claim of "research proven," they should have no problem supplying that information right? Wrong. My calls to many companies either yielded a mish-mash of junk science or nothing at all. One guy said to me "hey man, it's a marketing term" and quickly got off the phone. You would not believe what passes for "research" with some companies.

The real harm here is that good companies that do shell out the money for genuine research have to compete with companies that simply pretend to, and that can put the good companies at a real disadvantage, not to mention it fools people into potentially buying a product with no research at all behind it.

Used for thousands of years

Another gem of a marketing term! So if the product has only been used for 300 years, is it no good? People have also been eating things like tiger penis for thousands of years, does that mean it works or is safe? The answer is (drum roll).. No!

Of course at one time the earth was considered flat and it was once believed the sun revolved around the earth, but times change. Sure, an herb being used for a few thousand years, such as ephedra (Ma Huang) does lend some legitimacy to its safety and effectiveness, but it's far from proof the herb in question is either safe or effective. The bottom line here is that people have been using all sorts of things for thousands of years, some good, some not so good, some safe, some not so safe.

The term should not drive anyone to buy a product and assume that because it's been used for a thousand years (and remember we are assuming the company is even telling the truth about that) then it's safe and effective.

Proprietary Blend

In many cases, this is the most potentially misleading term of them all. While it doesn't always show up in the ads, it appears on the side of the bottle where it's used to reinforce the notion that the supplement ingredients are "scientifically formulated." It implies that the ingredients and amounts have been fine-tuned to work synergistically, and will produce better results than other brands, even ones using the same—or similar—ingredients.

Proprietary blends are not necessarily negative, though they are inherently confusing for the buyer in most cases.

A manufacturer will put the words "proprietary blend" on the label for one of two reasons:

- to prevent the competition from knowing exactly what ratios and amounts of each ingredient present in the formula, and to prevent the competition from copying their formula exactly (commonly referred to as a 'knock off') or

- to hide the fact the formula contains very little of the active ingredients listed on the bottle in an attempt to fool consumers.

What Label Decoration Means

Sadly where proprietary blends are concerned, the latter use is far more common than the former. A consumer will see a long list of seemingly impressive ingredients listed in the "proprietary blend" of a supplement, but in reality the things listed are such minute amounts that they don't have any effect.

This is commonly referred to as "label decoration" by industry insiders. The former use of the term is a legitimate way for a company of a quality formula from having the competition copy or "knock off" their formula and the latter use of the term is to scam people.

So how does the consumer tell the difference?

They can't, or at least they can't without some research and knowledge, which the scam artists know few people have the time and energy to dedicate to finding the answers. Although there are a few tips the consumer can use to decide if a product with a "proprietary blend" is worth trying, no one, not even me, can figure out exactly how much of each ingredient is in the blend or in what ratio of each is contained within the formula, hence why the honest and not so honest companies employ "proprietary blends" so often....

Well there you have it; my down and dirty guide to the world of marketing terms employed by some companies to sell products. As I alluded to above, these marketing tactics harm the legitimate companies out there trying to sell you a quality product by confusing the buyer who buys into the outlandish claims.

As always, the Latin expression "caveat emptor!" or "let the buyer beware" always applies.

HOW THIS BOOK WORKS

In the following pages, I've reviewed the claims and evidence for many of the most common compounds used in over-the-counter (OTC) diet supplements. I knew it would be simply impossible for me to review all of brand name supplements as any reviews I wrote would be rendered useless by changes in ingredients or recommended doses, and with new supplements constantly appearing on the market, this book would be obsolete within months.

This is why this book is focused on the ingredients in the supplements rather than the brand name supplements themselves, as these ingredients tend to be used over and over again, with exceptions to some of the new whiz-bang ingredients that are flashes in the pan from time to time.

An often used proverb goes *"Give a man a fish and you feed him for a day. Teach a man to fish and you feed him for a lifetime"*.

I put together this book in this manner to put the power of knowledge in your hands so that you can pick up any product and decide for yourself whether or not a particular brand name supplement is worth spending your hard earned money on.

Each review is broken into precise, easy to read sections. I've made all attempts not to put you to sleep with a lot of overly technical jargon, though it does exist in some sections of this book.

The sections are:

- ➤ **What is it?**
- ➤ **What is it supposed to do?**
- ➤ **What does the research say?**

> ➢ **What does the real world say for weight loss?**
> ➢ **Will Brink's Recommendation**

What is it? Will explain briefly what the compound is made of, where it comes from, and other pertinent information.

What is it supposed to do? Covers what a nutrient is supposed to do and how it achieves the effect, assuming it has an effect.

What does the research say? This is one of the more technical sections and will briefly look at the studies and sum up the research on a particular nutrient or formula where applicable.

What does the real world say for weight loss? Will sum up what people have said about their experience with each product. This section is a combination of the feedback I have received over the years and my own first hand experience with the many people I have worked with.

Of course, there's no particular formula or hard science behind this section but many readers may find it the most useful part of the book.

Will Brink's Recommendation Gives a summarization of the potential pros and cons of all the sections and give no B.S. advice on whether a product is worth using.

At the end of this book, I've also provided a **Weight Loss Supplements Scorecard** that summarizes the compounds that my research and experience have demonstrated are the most effective for fat loss.

Many of the compounds that I rate as "not worth the money" actually have positive effects on overall health—but if they don't help peel off the pounds, they don't make the cut on the Scorecard.

The Scorecard is followed by **How to Use the Weight Loss Supplement Scorecard** to analyze commercial supplements.

L–CARNITINE

What is it?

L–carnitine is an amino acid-like substance the body synthesizes from the amino acid lysine. The vitamins B–6, niacin, C, iron and the amino acid methionine are required for production of carnitine in the body.

The major dietary source of carnitine comes from animal meats, especially red meats (i.e. steak from cows, lamb and sheep).

Carnitine has many functions in the human body, but is best known for its ability to shuttle long chain fatty acids across the membrane of cells so they can be burned (oxidized) for energy by the mitochondria.

Mitochondria are often referred to as the "power house" of cells where energy is produced. The actual process of how carnitine shuttles fatty acids to the mitochondria is fairly complex and detailed. Suffice to say, it involves several enzymes and steps before the fats you want to burn end up being utilized by the mitochondria.

So, the carnitine shuttle system is essential for the body to be able to burn fats as energy, and this information can be found in any decent biochemistry text book.

What is it supposed to do?

As the above section mentions, carnitine is sold in hopes that it will help the body shuttle more fatty acids into cells to be used as energy rather than stored as abdominal-blurring blubber. The idea is that taking in

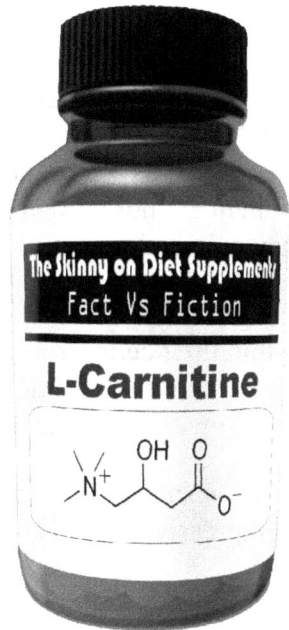

19

additional carnitine will supposedly help the body burn more fat for energy and make dieting more effective.

Carnitine is also sold as a sports supplement for increasing energy and may have several medical uses. The concept is pretty straightforward, but does it actually work?

What does the research say?

Studies that have focused on weight loss in people using carnitine as a supplement are few and conflicting. There are far more studies that look at carnitine as a sport and energy enhancing supplement, but the majority of them are not very impressive, although some studies suggest carnitine may help endurance athletes.

The general consensus is that healthy people have plenty of carnitine within their cells (from the body's own production and dietary intake) for the carnitine shuttle system to work, though it has been shown that very low calorie diets do alter carnitine metabolism.

The few studies that have looked at weight loss with carnitine have been unimpressive.

For example, a study that looked at 36 moderately overweight women given 4 grams of carnitine per day for 60 days—using a double blind placebo protocol—found no significant changes in any of the end points examined (i.e., body weight, LBM, and fat oxidation).

What does the real world say for weight loss?

In the real world, feedback on carnitine for weight loss has been generally disappointing. I have yet to find anyone who has lost weight due to the simple addition of carnitine to their diet.

Will Brink's Recommendation

Carnitine is a perfect example of a supplement, as mentioned in the introduction to this book, that is useful for some applications but not for others.

In people with serious metabolic problems where fatty acid metabolism has been altered, carnitine has been shown to be of clinical use. Carnitine is even listed in the *Physicians Desk Reference* (a.k.a. "the PDR") for certain pathologies involving the heart, and many alternative doctors swear by it for that use.

Carnitine may also help reduce cholesterol and increase HDL ("good") cholesterol. Carnitine is a very safe supplement with no known toxic effects.

Although it may very well have potential health benefits in certain people, the bottom line is that it does not appear to be all that effective as a weight loss nutrient.

It is also quite an expensive supplement and companies will add very small amounts for label decoration.

If you want to use carnitine, you will need to use at least 500 mg or more several times daily (some studies have used 5000-6000 mg or more daily).

If you see 20, 50, or 100 mg of carnitine in some weight loss formula, it's nothing but label decoration and will have little effect.

Considering the cost, the amount needed for an effect, and the lack of solid research regarding weight loss, carnitine gets a poor rating in my book for weight loss, though it may have its health uses. Carnitine is one of those ingredients that fool people into thinking it's an effective weight loss agent, for reasons that are unclear.

Food Sources of Carnitine

L-Carnitine Content of Selected Foods		
Food	**Serving**	**L-Carnitine (mg)**
Beef steak	3 ounces*	81
Ground beef	3 ounces	80
Pork	3 ounces	24
Canadian bacon	3 ounces	20
Milk (whole)	8 fluid ounces (1 cup)	8
Fish (cod)	3 ounces	5
Chicken breast	3 ounces	3
Ice cream	4 ounces (1/2 cup)	3
Avocado	1 medium	2
American cheese	1 ounce	1
Whole-wheat bread	2 slices	0.2
Asparagus	6 spears (1/2 cup)	0.2

*A 3-ounce serving of meat is about the size of a deck of cards.

Source: Linus Pauling Institute
http://lpi.oregonstate.edu/infocenter/othernuts/carnitine/

ACETYL–L–CARNITINE

What is it?

Acetyl–L–Carnitine (ALC), as the name implies, is related to carnitine. ALC has many functions in the human body that differ from carnitine, but in essence, they are the same compound from a practical point of view.

What is it supposed to do?

Specific to weight loss, the reader can think of ALC as similar L-Carnitine.

What does the research say?

The research on ALC relating to weight loss is even more lacking than with carnitine. Research with ALC has generally focused on its potential health benefits, of which there are many. ALC does have some unique differences from that of carnitine, but those differences don't appear to have any added effects on weight loss per se.

What does the real world say for weight loss?

Pretty much the same thing as carnitine; for weight loss it's a bust as far as feedback is concerned.

Will Brink's Recommendation

You don't have to be a mind reader to know what I am going to say about ALC and weight loss.

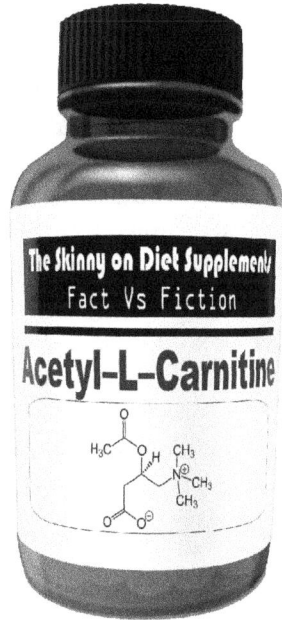

It's even more expensive than carnitine, has even less research behind it (as it relates to weight loss), and the feedback has generally been negative. However, like carnitine, ALC has many health uses and is very safe, which is why researchers and the medical community have taken a real interest in ALC.

ALC has been shown to have protective effects on the brain and heart tissue during low oxygen states from lack of blood flow (known as ischemia) and is of particular interest for mental functions associated with aging. It may also lower cholesterol and raise HDL.

It's often sold as a sports supplement because some animal research suggests it may raise testosterone, but the research on that is very much lacking and inconclusive. More recent studies have found ALC, and other forms of Carnitine, may improve endurance, but again, studies have been mixed and doses needed to get the effect, quite high.

So, for various health uses, ALC is very promising stuff. For weight loss, there are far better ways to spend your money. Typical doses range widely, from 1g (1000 mg) to 5-6 g or more.

CAYENNE (CAPSAICIN)

What is it?

Cayenne is a spice made from dried, ground chili peppers. In foods, it contributes a hot, spicy taste due to its content of capsaicin (See also piperine section for additional info).

What is it supposed to do?

A certain amount of food energy you eat is used to fuel the processes of digestion and absorption. This energy requirement is known as the "thermic effect of food" or "diet-induced thermogenesis" (DIT). Consuming cayenne or capsicum may increase DIT and fat oxidation, particularly after a high fat meal.

So, in theory, using cayenne may help you burn off some additional calories that might otherwise end up on your butt.

What does the research say?

Experiments with rats and mice have demonstrated that capsaicin administration can enhance thermogenesis (i.e., increase the number of calories burned), and—at high (100 mg/kg) doses—improve glucose tolerance. Human experiments suggest that the thermogenic response is relatively weak, however.

One study measured an increase in energy expenditure of only 200 kJ (less than 50 kcal) after using a supplement containing capsaicin.

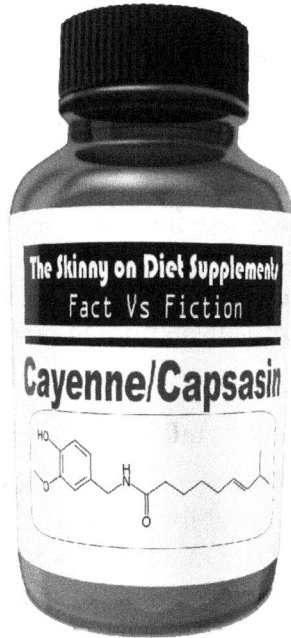

In another recent study, "**Sensory and gastrointestinal satiety effects of capsaicin on food intake**" subjects ate less when 900 mg capsaicin was taken before a meal. The greatest increase in satiety and decrease in calorie intake occurred when the capsaicin was mixed in tomato juice vs. taken in capsules. This implies a sensory effect was involved as well.

Capsaicin–induced increases in DIT may be reduced in obesity. When a capsaicin-containing meal was given to obese women, the thermogenic response was lower than in lean women consuming the same meal.

What does the real world say for weight loss?

Capsaicin also exerts local effects on the gastrointestinal tract, and increases intestinal permeability (*J Nutr*. 1998 Mar;128(3):577–81.). The downside of this is that taking capsaicin could increase the potential for developing allergies to specific foods or food components. The same probably applies to piperine, by the way (see section on Piperine).

Will Brink's Recommendation

I have some reservations about cayenne/capsaicin, due to the intestinal permeability issue; over the long–term, having a "leaky gut" is not a good thing. People with known pre-existing leaky gut syndrome should probably avoid cayenne/capsaicin supplements, but there's essentially no data to go on there.

In my opinion, capsaicin or cayenne are probably best used as seasonings in food, which appears to be the best way to take advantage of capsaicin's ability to enhance satiety.

There appears to be very little benefit to taking it in supplement form for weight loss. If not followed by a meal afterward, taking this supplement on an empty stomach can give you one heck of a case of heartburn. I found that out the hard way myself once.

CHITOSAN

What is it?

Chitosan is technically a fiber which is derived from the tough outer layer of shellfish. It was originally manufactured for water treatment applications as it binds to heavy metals, oils, and other pollutants.

What is it supposed to do?

Chitosan works primarily through positive and negative charge interactions. Translated, chitosan has a positive charge which attracts negatively charged materials such as lipids (fats).

If a person takes chitosan with a high fat meal, the fat will (hopefully) bind to the chitosan during digestion and will be excreted from the body before it is ever absorbed, so it can't be stored as body fat.

Manufacturers of chitosan claim it can bind up to eight times its weight in fat, but it's probably more like five to six times. Chitosan may also have health uses for people with high cholesterol levels.

What does the research say?

As might be expected from a product of this nature, research has mainly focused on the possible effects of chitosan on cholesterol and triglyceride levels. Animal and human studies suggest chitosan is an effective reducer of cholesterol and triglycerides, with some studies showing a rise in HDL ("good") cholesterol and a reduction in LDL ("bad") cholesterol.

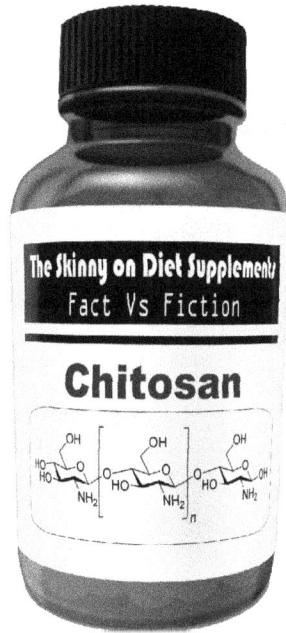

One study found men using up to 6 grams daily of chitosan had an 11 point drop in total cholesterol and an increase in HDL in just two weeks. Higher amounts in animals—up to 5% of the animal's diet—showed even more impressive drops in cholesterol levels with increases in HDL levels.

As its industrial use would imply, chitosan binds to the fat, cholesterol, and bile, which not being available for absorption; is simply excreted. As for weight loss, several small studies appeared to show a statistically significant improvement on weight loss with chitosan, while another larger and more recent study found no effect. The difference may have been in the dosage between the different studies.

As with carnitine and CLA, the effective dose is probably much higher than what is found on the bottle of most products.

What does the real world say for weight loss?

Strangely, though chitosan has been sold for several years, I have gotten very little feedback about this product. What little feedback I have gotten has been mixed, so I can't give a clear and useful picture regarding the real world opinion or "buzz" on chitosan at this time.

Will Brink's Recommendation

Personally I have many qualms with products such as chitosan that work by blocking the uptake of dietary fats.

Why?

Many essential nutrients important to our health are found in fats, including the fat-soluble vitamins E, A, D, and K, and blocking the absorption of fats with chitosan could potentially lead to deficiencies in these and other nutrients.

As chitosan blocks the absorption of fats, it might also block the uptake of the essential fatty acids (EFAs) we all need for optimal health and weight loss (see section on EFAs for more info).

Chitosan may also reduce the absorption of minerals, and one study showed mineral absorption and bone density was reduced in animals fed chitosan.

Related to the fat–soluble vitamin issue, the same study also found a

"marked and rapid decrease in the serum vitamin E level..."

Other animal studies have shown a blunting of growth with high amounts of chitosan. When a deficiency in any of the above nutrients could negatively affect long term health, I have to question the wisdom of long term use of chitosan.

Chitosan might be a moderately useful part of a total plan to lose fat, but it would be a mistake for a person to rely on it as their sole method of weight loss.

So what's the take home message on chitosan?

It might be an effective aid in reducing cholesterol and triglycerides. It might also be an aid to weight loss, if used as a small part of the weight loss arsenal available to people. In this writer's opinion there are better ways to safely lose weight.

Of course, some people are bound to be attracted to the idea of blocking fat absorption and will use it regardless of these warnings as they have been brainwashed into believing fat is bad.

The best advice at this time for people interested in using chitosan would be to use it for specific periods of dieting (e.g., 8-12 weeks), and take additional fat-soluble vitamins, minerals, and essential fatty acids at least 3-4 hours apart from the chitosan to address any potential deficiencies that might occur.

Oh, here's a tip when using chitosan: chitosan forms a gel with the fats, bile and cholesterol, which is then excreted. It has been found that adding vitamin C to chitosan appears to further enhance the formation of the gel.

So, adding, say, 100-200 mg of vitamin C to the chitosan (both of which should be taken 30-40 minutes prior to a meal with a large glass of water) may improve its effects.

Alternate Dietary Forms of Fiber

Description	Weight (g)	Common Measure	Content per Measure (grams)
Barley, pearled, raw	200	1 cup	31.2
Bulgur, dry	140	1 cup	25.6
Beans, navy, mature seeds, cooked, boiled, without salt	182	1 cup	19.1
Peas, split, mature seeds, cooked, boiled, without salt	196	1 cup	16.3
Lentils, mature seeds, cooked, boiled, without salt	198	1 cup	15.6
Beans, pinto, mature seeds, cooked, boiled, without salt	171	1 cup	15.4
Beans, black, mature seeds, cooked, boiled, without salt	172	1 cup	15
Oat bran, raw	94	1 cup	14.5
Artichokes, (globe or french), cooked, boiled, drained, without salt	168	1 cup	14.4
Dates, deglet noor	178	1 cup	14.2
Beans, kidney, red, mature seeds, canned, solids and liquids	256	1 cup	13.6
Lima beans, large, mature seeds, cooked, boiled, without salt	188	1 cup	13.2
Beans, kidney, red, mature seeds, cooked, boiled, without salt	177	1 cup	13.1
Wheat flour, whole-grain	120	1 cup	12.8
Beans, white, mature seeds, canned	262	1 cup	12.6
Chickpeas (garbanzo beans, bengal gram), mature seeds, cooked, boiled, without salt	164	1 cup	12.5
Beans, great northern, mature seeds, cooked, boiled, without salt	177	1 cup	12.4

source: USDA Agricultural Research Service
http://www.ars.usda.gov/Services/docs.htm?docid=22114

CHROMIUM

What is it?

Chromium is a mineral essential to blood sugar metabolism, as well as other important functions related to insulin and fat metabolism.

What is it supposed to do?

As insulin is a primary fat storage hormone in the human body, it is presumed anything that improves the actions of insulin will help prevent weight gain and food cravings.

It has been well established that chromium, along with other nutrients, is essential for proper insulin functioning.

Chromium supplements usually come as chromium picolinate, but can also be found as chromium polynicotinate, a form some studies suggest is superior to the picolinate form.

Some studies suggest chromium can help reduce cholesterol levels and triglyceride levels and improve HDL levels, which would make perfect sense considering this mineral's role in blood sugar and lipid metabolism. Some feel it's also useful for people with blood sugar management problems, such as hypoglycemia.

What does the research say?

Traditionally, companies marketing chromium tend to heavily emphasize research that demonstrated chromium could help with fat loss and increases in lean body mass (LBM).

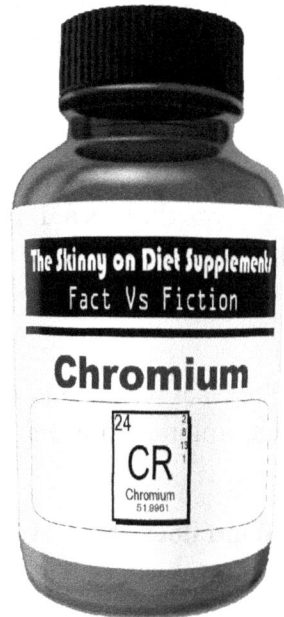

31

Early studies gave glowing reports on chromium and showed significant reductions in body fat and increases in muscle when given to college aged athletes. This research was criticized for having extensive flaws, however.

As recently as 1997, no fewer than six studies using various populations ranging from old to young subjects, showed chromium supplementation had no effect on muscle mass or body fat. In fact, one study found that older women (age range 54-71) given high doses of chromium and put on a strength training regimen gained less muscle than the group that didn't receive the supplement!

On the flip side, a more recent study looks very promising for chromium as a weight loss aid. In the study, 122 overweight people who were given 400 mcg of chromium picolinate for 90 days lost over six pounds of body fat. This was almost twice what the placebo group lost in body fat.

So, what we have is conflicting research regarding the effects of chromium and weight loss.

What does the real world have to say for weight loss?

Just like the feedback on carnitine, chromium looks good on paper, but has been unimpressive in the real world. I have not seen anyone lose weight at an increased rate due to the simple addition of chromium to their diet, nor has anyone at any of my seminars or radio shows, ever really raved about chromium for fat loss.

Will Brink's Recommendation

After reading the information presented above, how do we come to grips with all the conflicting research on chromium as a product used for weight loss?

Its well known that exercise, diets high in sugar, and other factors drain the body's stores of chromium. It's also fairly well established that a large proportion of Americans don't get enough chromium in their diets, as much of the food people eat has been stripped of its chromium by modern processing techniques.

32

Finally, we know that chromium is an essential nutrient to human health and is critical for the regulation of proper blood sugar metabolism.

Clearly, chromium is a nutrient that we should strive to get from a good supplement and/or from our food. There is no doubt that people deficient in chromium will get positive effects from ingesting chromium whether or not they lose weight.

Whether people who are not deficient will get any effect from additional chromium as you can tell by some of the studies, is also questionable.

To view chromium as a miracle fat loss supplement or ergogenic sports aid is premature. You should make sure you get sufficient chromium in your diet from a variety of sources (i.e., multivitamin/mineral supplement, whole grains, various weight loss formulas, etc.), but extra isn't needed.

Chromium is perfectly safe at normal recommended intakes found in most supplements. However, in extremely high doses—above 1000 mcg or more per day for long periods of time—chromium can be toxic.

General advice for people who want to use chromium supplements is to use 300-600 micrograms (mcg) per day.

Syndrome X: What it is, how to combat it

Chromium, and other nutrients, may be useful in a common health problem known as Syndrome X. Some studies suggest Syndrome X:

- Afflicts 70-80 million people, almost one third of Americans
- Is linked to obesity and weight gain
- Is associated with diabetes
- Is associated with high blood pressure
- Is a common factor in cardiovascular disease and stroke
- Is a primary cause of a lowered metabolism and fatigue

The term Syndrome X is actually a description for insulin resistance and all the potential pathologies that can come with it (i.e. obesity, reduced metabolism, cardiovascular disease, etc.).

Insulin resistance was dubbed "Syndrome X" in 1988 because it's found along with so many different medical conditions.

In other parts of the world there are various terms for insulin resistance. One such term is C.H.A.O.S, which is short for "Coronary heart disease, Hypertension/hyperlipidemia, Adult-onset diabetes, Obesity, and Stroke." Ouch!

Another term for the same syndrome is "Insulin Resistance Metabolic Syndrome" or IRMS for short. Today, IRMS is simply referred to as "Metabolic Syndrome."

All over the world the scientific and medical community is starting to see that many seemingly unrelated diseases are in fact linked to a malfunction in insulin and/or blood sugar metabolism. Insulin resistance can underlie these various illnesses because the hormone insulin plays such an important and pivotal role in the body.

Among its hundreds of different functions, the body uses insulin to control the amount of sugar (glucose) in the blood, help pull amino acids into the cells, turn on protein synthesis in lean tissues, and regulate body fat storage.

Problems with the body's ability to regulate blood glucose appear if insulin does not properly bind to its receptors on the membranes of the cells or if, for other reasons, blood sugar is not readily accepted by the cells.

As already indicated, insulin resistance is the general name for the failure of normal amounts of insulin to maintain blood sugar (i.e., glucose). When insulin does not bring blood sugar down after meals, the body secretes even higher amounts of insulin until serum glucose levels eventually fall.

Insulin resistance has several possible causes, including the over-consumption of simple and refined carbohydrates and/or a lack of adequate nutrients combined with genetic factors. Of course the heavy

34

over consumption of processed simple carbohydrates coupled with inadequate nutrient intake is a mainstay of the American diet.

Conversely, and not surprisingly, diets and nutrients which reduce the amount of insulin required by the body also appear to reduce the tendency toward excessive weight gain.

Inasmuch as the hormone insulin is well known for its ability to store glucose in muscle, increase protein synthesis, and possibly increase muscle mass, it has predictably gotten the attention of bodybuilders and other athletes. In fact, it is sometimes said that insulin is the primary anabolic hormone produced by the body.

Some researchers feel that insulin is, in fact, more important to lean muscle tissue than the better known anabolic hormones testosterone and growth hormone (GH).

Unfortunately, insulin certainly has its downsides. Of course most people know that out of control insulin metabolism will make a person rather fat, since insulin is a primary hormonal mediator of fat storage. Insulin resistance increases the number of calories stored as fat and increases the amount of fat produced by the liver from carbohydrates.

And it gets worse; it turns out that insulin plays a big role in whether we produce our own fat from carbohydrates. And if we are making even a little fat, we turn off our ability to burn fat because the body does not make new fat and burn already stored fat at the same time.

Of course the concept of "insulin management" for adding new muscle to the hard training athlete's frame is all the rage with various bodybuilding magazines, supplement companies, and nutritional guru types. If you can manage insulin correctly, you can add new muscle without adding a great deal of body fat, and this has been the goal of proper insulin management.

It's obvious that athletes and bodybuilders are far more aware than the general public of the importance of insulin, hence the popularity of insulin-potentiating minerals such as chromium and vanadyl sulfate.

Of course, some bodybuilders have chosen to go the Kamikaze route by injecting insulin directly, but it does not take a rocket scientist to realize how dangerous this practice is.

Can you say "coma?"

Also, many bodybuilders who play with insulin injections end up looking more like the "Michelin Man" than a bodybuilder.

One thing should be clear by now: proper insulin management is of paramount importance both for athletes looking to add new muscle without adding body fat as well as non-athletes trying to avoid a host of medical ills.

Athletes want to improve their insulin/blood sugar metabolism because they know it can lead to increases in lean mass, glycogen storage in muscle, and decreases in body fat. Avoiding future medical problems is certainly not a bad motivator either.

On the plus side for bodybuilders and exercise buffs in general, regular exercise improves insulin sensitivity. On the nutritional side, fiber and nutrients such as vitamin C, E, magnesium, omega–3 fatty acids (see sections on fish/flax oils), and chromium have been shown to improve glucose metabolism.

Diabetics, people with Syndrome X, and athletes who want to improve insulin metabolism/insulin sensitivity would be wise to include these nutrients in their diets.

Whether you're a bodybuilder, runner, general fitness buff, or average Joe/Jane, understanding insulin metabolism and what happens when it goes haywire is essential for gaining muscle, losing body fat, and avoiding the spiral into disease that is Syndrome X.

Avoiding Syndrome X, and the many diseases associated with it, is a matter of regular exercise, adequate and correct nutrient intake, avoiding health degrading substances, and using some common sense. Too bad we don't have a common sense pill yet!

Dietary Sources of Chromium

Food	Chromium Content (mcg)
Broccoli, ½ cup	11
Grape juice, 1 cup	8
English muffin, whole wheat, 1	4
Potatoes, mashed, 1 cup	3
Garlic, dried, 1 teaspoon	3
Basil, dried, 1 tablespoon	2
Beef cubes, 3 ounces	2
Orange juice, 1 cup	2
Turkey breast, 3 ounces	2
Whole wheat bread, 2 slices	2
Red wine, 5 ounces	1–13
Apple, unpeeled, 1 medium	1
Banana, 1 medium	1
Green beans, ½ cup	1

Possible Drug Interactions to be aware of

Medications	Nature of interaction
Antacids Corticosteroids H2 blockers (such as cimetidine, famotidine, nizatidine, and rantidine) Proton-pump inhibitors (such as omeprazole, lansoprazole, rabeprazole, pantoprazole, and esomeprazole)	These medications alter stomach acidity and may impair chromium absorption or enhance excretion

Medications	Nature of interaction
Beta-blockers (such as atenolol or propanolol) Corticosteroids Insulin Nicotinic acid Nonsteroidal anti-inflammatory drugs (NSAIDS) Prostaglandin inhibitors (such as ibuprofen, indomethacin, naproxen, piroxicam, and aspirin)	These medications may have their effects enhanced if taken together with chromium or they may increase chromium absorption

Source:
http://ods.od.nih.gov/factsheets/chromium/

CITRUS AURANTIUM /SYNEPHRINE

What is it?

Synephrine is derived from Citrus aurantium, a.k.a, bitter orange or zhi shi. Synephrine is quite similar in chemical structure to compounds such as ephedrine (see ephedrine/caffeine section for a description of ephedrine) and pseudoephedrine, which makes it a stimulant and beta–agonist.

What is it supposed to do?

Companies selling synephrine frequently make the claim it has the same metabolic effects as ephedrine and other beta–agonists (i.e. increased metabolic rate, weight loss, etc.) but without the side effects of ephedrine. Although Citrus aurantium extracts contain synephrine, they also contain other potentially active compounds such as N–methyltyramine, hordenine, octopamine and tyramine.

Companies make this claim about synephrine because the active compounds in Citrus aurantium stimulate only beta–3 receptors; not the beta–1, or beta–2 receptors; so the negative effects of ephedrine and other stimulants are avoided while metabolic rate is increased.

Beta–3 receptors are concentrated in what is called "brown adipose tissue" or BAT, which is more metabolically active than "regular" white fat and is involved in metabolic rate and other functions, though beta–3 receptors are expressed in much lower amounts in both muscle and white fat.

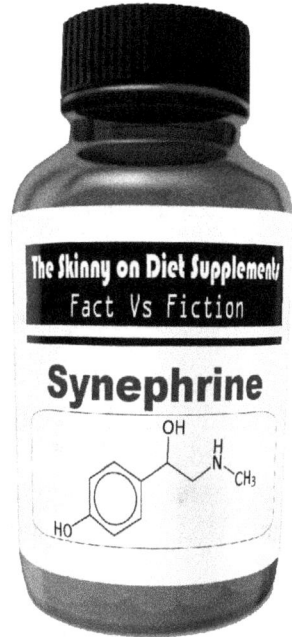

BAT differs from white fat not just in color. BAT has a large number of mitochondria (the part of the cell where energy is produced) that contain something called "uncoupling protein," which can stimulate oxidative phosphorylation and thereby increase metabolic rate. BAT is present to oxidize lipids (i.e., burn fat) in order to produce heat and rid the body of excess adipose tissue (i.e., blubber, fat, lard, or what ever you want to call it).

Let's get a bit more technical for those of you who are interested;

Agonizing (stimulating) the beta–3 receptor found in BAT, activates the enzyme adenylate cyclase, which increases intracellular concentrations of cyclic AMP and results in increase lipolysis and thermogenesis.

As one might expect, many big name pharmaceutical companies have also pursued beta–3 agonists as possible weight loss drugs.

For example, Ciba-Geigy had at least one drug, code name GCP 12177, Sanofi-Midy has an other code named SR 58611A, ICI Labs had at least two, code named ICI D7114 and ICI 215001, and Smith-Kline Beecham had at least four, code named BRL 26830A, BRL 37344, BRL 49653, and BRL 35135 respectively.

Other companies have also looked into developing specific beta–3 agonist compounds for the multi-billion dollar weight loss market, but to date, nothing has come to market for that use.

What does the research have to say?

Because beta–3 agonists were found to simultaneously increase lipolysis, fat oxidation, energy expenditure, and insulin action in animals, this led to the belief that this receptor might serve as an attractive target for the treatment of diabetes and obesity. Research has been intense.

One investigation, **"Potentiations of the anti-obesity effect of the selective beta–3 adrenoreceptor agonist BRL 35135 in obese Zucker rats by exercise"** (*Br J Pharm*. 1994 Dec; 113(4): 1231–6), gave BRL 35135 (a beta–3 agonist) at a dose of 0.5 mg/kg orally to half the rats in the study while the other half got a placebo (I don't know why they would give animals a placebo…)

Body weight, food intake, brown adipose tissue thermogenesis and plasma insulin/glucose levels were measured in both groups after 3 weeks of treatment. The rats that received the beta–3 agonist showed a 45-fold increase in brown fat thermogenic activity, and a decrease in plasma insulin levels of 50%. The effect of the drug was significantly enhanced by exercise; the reduction in weight gain was 56% compared to 19% in sedentary animals.

Another journal article, **"Clinical studies with the beta–adrenoreceptor agonist BRL 26830A"** (*Am J Clin Nutr*. 1992 Jan; 55(1): 258S–261S) discusses a double-blind study with 40 obese patients who received either BRL 26830A or a placebo for 18 weeks. Both groups were put on a calorie-restricted diet.

After 18 weeks, the BRL 26830A group had a weight loss of 33.88 lbs. (median) while the control group had a median weight loss of only 22 lbs. Urinary nitrogen excretion was similar in both groups which suggested that the weight loss was mainly from adipose tissue, not muscle.

Psychological assessments showed that BRL 26830A had no adverse effects in mood, hunger, or satiety, which seems odd as most beta–agonists usually suppress hunger. Most people who take drugs such as Clenbuterol or OTC beta–agonists such as ephedrine notice a reduction in hunger.

Of course it should be noted that this effect was found with a synthetic drug.

Even more important to note is that although there have been some impressive studies; there have also been some spectacular failures in this area of drug development. Major obstacles have included the pharmacological differences between the rodent and human beta–3 receptors, poor oral bioavailability of the drugs as well as other problems.

So far, this area of drug development has had a very rocky start.

Specific to synephrine/Citrus aurantium, studies in animals have suggested an increased metabolic rate and a decrease in food intake in animals given the extracts from Citrus aurantium. There have been a limited number of studies that were done in humans using extracts of Citrus aurantium, but they have suffered from serious methodological flaws and/or were done as a combination formula containing other herbs, making it impossible to tell exactly what caused the weight loss.

Also, some studies indicate the effects/mechanism of synephrine may be that it acts as a vasodilator rather than a true thermogenic compound. A vasodilator might make you feel hot to the touch (because of the increased blood flow to the skin) but you are not burning more calories via thermogenesis.

What does the real world say for weight loss?

Feedback to date has been moderate to negative with most people reporting little or no effect. Some do report a reduced appetite. Also, as mentioned above, Citrus aurantium generally comes mixed with other herbs and other compounds in a formula rather than sold as single ingredient, so it's near impossible to separate the effects of the Citrus aurantium over the other ingredients.

Will Brink's Recommendation

So far, I have not been impressed with this herb for weight loss. The studies done to date that found any effects on weight loss always had it combined with other herbs, so no real conclusion can be made. Studies done alone are mixed and or not very impressive though it may be a mild appetite suppressant.

It bothers me that companies who are selling the products claim it stimulates beta–3 cell receptors with minimal effect on other alpha and beta receptors. This would mean that Citrus aurantium "increases metabolic rate without affecting heart rate or blood pressure" to quote one company.

There is one very major flaw to this statement; rats and mice have large areas of fat that are exclusively made of BAT to help them regulate body temperature, body fat levels, and other important metabolic functions, and newborn human babies also have distinct areas of brown fat, but adult humans don't have a lot of distinct brown adipose tissue.

At this point, I consider Citrus aurantium/synephrine as far more hype due to the lack of solid credible studies showing effects in humans.

As for dose, 4-20 mg of synephrine per day is a typical dose found in products providing 200-600 mg of a standardized Citrus aurantium extract (3-6% synephrine). As for safety, I think companies pushing it as totally without side effects are misleading the public.

Studies have shown both the herb and the synthetic versions can raise blood pressure at high enough doses, but no studies have found any acute toxicity at normal doses.

Who should __not__ take this stuff

Because synephrine/Citrus aurantium is a stimulant, you should not take without consulting a physician if you have any of the following conditions:

- If you don't tolerate stimulants well.

- Have pre-existing medical conditions such as heart disease have any heart irregularities or high blood pressure.

- Are taking MAOI inhibitors.

- If you have prostate disease.

- If you are pregnant.

Mixing different stimulants (e.g., ephedrine and theophylline, etc.) could increase the potential for side effects above what is acceptable.

If using any of the above stimulants in conjunction with EC products,

I would recommend cutting back on the dose of EC to account for the additional effects of these other stimulants.

CONJUGATED LINOLEIC ACID (CLA)

What is it?

Conjugated linoleic acid (CLA) is a fatty acid derived from the essential fatty acid linoleic acid. CLA is found predominantly in dairy products and some meats and appears to be a fat with some unique effects on the metabolism of animals and (hopefully) people.

What is it supposed to do?

CLA has been sold as both a fat loss supplement and as a sports nutrition product for adding muscle. The sellers of CLA focus on the fact that in animals such as rats and mice, CLA causes rats and mice to lose body fat while adding lean tissue (i.e., muscle).

Like so many products, CLA may have legitimate health uses. CLA can be found as different isomers (i.e., cis–9,trans–11 and trans–10,cis–12 isomers) and recent research suggests different isomers are responsible for different effects, such as anticancer, anti-obesity, etc.

What does the research say?

CLA has been found to be the best thing for mice and rats since they slipped anabolic steroids in their mouse food! A substantial number of studies have confirmed that animals (the aforementioned squeaky things with red eyes) add lean body mass (muscle) and lose body fat when fed CLA, making CLA a true anabolic agent in rodents.

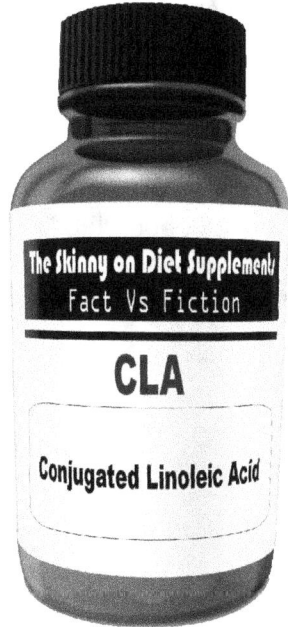

"Ok," you're thinking, "lots of things work on mice and rats but don't seem to do a thing for us higher animals who want to lose fat." That is true, and like many supplements sold as weight loss agents, the human data is lacking.

The few human studies that have been done are limited and produced mixed results. There was one interesting human study recently completed with bodybuilders. This research was presented by a Dr. Lowery at a large conference in Lahti, Finland.

The study fed 24 novice athletes 12 grams of a product containing 7.2 grams of CLA or a placebo (vegetable oil) while completing a 6 week program of bodybuilding exercises. The study found the group getting CLA had an increase in strength and arm girth (their arms got larger) but did not add body fat.

The researchers concluded

> *"... apparently, CLA acts as a mild anabolic agent in novice male bodybuilders."*

No doubt, this finding needs to be confirmed in a larger study.

The good news about CLA is there have been several new studies in humans. The bad news is they continue to be conflicting in their findings. For example, one recent study found that CLA supplementation at 3-4 grams per day caused an almost one inch reduction in waist size and a loss of body fat of 2-4 lbs in overweight subjects over a 12 week period.

However, a pilot study using weight lifters found no differences in body weight, fat, or muscle mass over a 30-day period. Another small study using 10 subjects receiving 3-4 grams of CLA vs. 10 subjects getting a placebo for three months, found similar results.

Still another study of 17 healthy women getting 3 grams of CLA vs. placebo (sunflower oil) for 64 days, found no statistically significant differences between the two groups.

What does the real world say for weight loss?

The general feedback on CLA has been mixed in regards to fat loss. There are some people who have reported that taken in high enough amounts, CLA seemed to help with fat loss. However, the majority of people I have spoken with, and all the people I have worked with on a one-on-one basis, reported no effects from using CLA.

Will Brink's Recommendation

The vast majority of research with CLA has been performed with animals (rats and mice), and we are not rats and mice, though new human studies have just recently popped up. The metabolism of rats and mice vs. people is often quite different regarding fats and carbohydrates, though this does not mean animal research should be ignored.

Some researchers feel there is a specific threshold intake of CLA needed to get an effect. For example, Dr. Lowery's study cited above used 7 grams of CLA a day.

Although it was a small study, the results were promising. On the other hand, 7 grams of CLA per day is an expensive proposition as the stuff is not cheap.

However, we now have a handful of studies using 3-4 grams that have come to conflicting conclusions, so you will have to make up their own mind on the importance of that finding.

Lesser amounts (such as a few hundred milligrams) of CLA often found in weight loss supplements are nothing but label decoration.

As for the health uses of CLA, several in-vitro (test tube) and animal studies have shown it has powerful antioxidant properties as well as impressive anticancer properties. It has been shown to modulate insulin–like growth factor binding proteins (IGFBPs) in mice and may also improve insulin sensitivity.

It has been shown to suppress the growth of certain lines of human breast cancer as well as several other cancers. Animals exposed to various cancer-causing chemicals and fed CLA fare much better than those not getting CLA. Some studies with CLA also point to this lipid as a possible immune enhancer.

CLA is also appears to be a very safe product.

The bottom line is, though CLA may turn out to be a worthwhile supplement for losing fat, far more human research is needed for definitive conclusions. I consider CLA a supplement to keep an eye on, but there are better and more cost effective options, especially considering the cost of CLA and the lack of—or conflicting—human data.

People interested in using CLA probably need at least 3 grams or more per day of CLA, as the human studies would suggest as the minimum effective dose, though 4-7 grams would probably be better.

Co–Enzyme Q10

What is it?

Co–enzyme Q10, or Q10 for short, is involved in energy production at the cellular level. Q10 is part of the electron transfer chain involved in the production of ATP. If that sounds confusing, it's not important to remember if you don't want to.

The body produces Q10 from the foods we eat, and the amino acid methionine is known to be important for its production. Foods such as organ meats and fish contain small amounts of Q10.

Like L–carnitine, Q10 works in the mitochondria to produce energy. It may have health benefits and is an antioxidant.

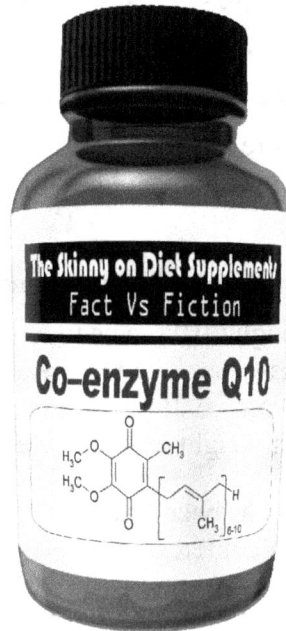

What is it supposed to do?

Q10 has been recommended to overweight people as a means of burning more calories by increasing energy production from food, rather than storing it as body fat, because it may improve energy production at the cellular level.

What does the research say?

The research looking at Q10 as a weight loss agent is nonexistent for all practical purposes. Interestingly however, some research found obese people are deficient in Q10.

What that means to weight loss is unknown, and companies who have recommended the use of Q10 based on that knowledge are taking a shot in the dark.

Q10 is used extensively in Japan, and other countries, as a treatment for certain heart conditions, especially congestive heart failure. Some studies suggest it can improve endurance. It may also improve immunity, but research on Q10 as a rule has been contradictory.

What does the real world say for weight loss?

If there is a human being in the world who has lost weight with Q10, I have yet to meet him or her.

Will Brink's Recommendation

Though Q10 seems to have various potential health benefits, proof that it has any use as a fat loss agent is very much lacking and less than impressive. It is also exceedingly expensive and the amounts found in most weight loss formulas would not affect a mouse much less a person.

Q10 has been found to be totally safe and has no known toxic effects. People interested in Q10 for health reasons, or who just want to take an expensive shot in the dark at weight loss, should take 25-100 mg or more daily.

Relating to its possible role in heart disease, alternative medical researchers "in the know" suggest Q10 be combined with carnitine, magnesium, and vitamin E for optimal effect.

DHEA

What is it?

Dehydroepiandrosterone (DHEA) is a hormone produced primarily in the adrenal glands with minor amounts produced by the testes. It is found in both men and women. DHEA is the most abundant steroid hormone in the human body, and like all steroid hormones, ultimately comes from cholesterol.

Most DHEA in the body is found as DHEA-sulfate (DHEA–S). DHEA is a major precursor to other steroid hormones, which is why some companies market it as a "muscle builder."

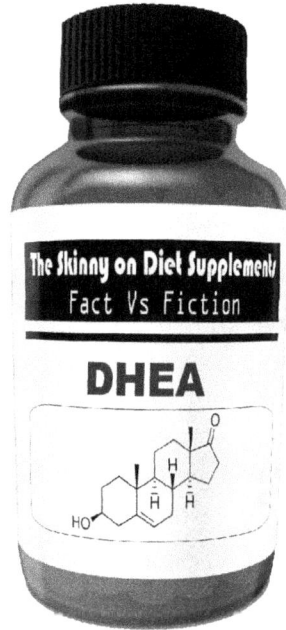

What is it supposed to do?

DHEA is marketed as being helpful for just about every human ailment from memory loss to heart disease to immune enhancement to weight loss, and more.

What does the research say?

DHEA consistently makes rodents such as mice and rats lose weight. In red eyed rodents (i.e. mice and rats), DHEA causes many biochemical changes that just don't seem to happen in people, showing just how different rats and people can be.

In people, the research has been far less impressive. Several studies using over 1500 mg per day of DHEA showed either no effects or short-lived effects on weight loss in humans.

One early study found 1600 mg per day of DHEA (a very high dose of DHEA) reduced body fat and increased muscle mass in men, with later studies done by the same group and others failing to find that effect. However, one recent study on DHEA found only 150 mg per day increased lean body mass in young men and increased IGF–1.

Some studies in people using DHEA have shown slight increases in testosterone and insulin–like growth factor 1 (IGF–1) levels, but most studies have found minimal effect in people.

The research showing health improvements, such as cognitive benefits, immune enhancement, stress reduction, and anticancer benefits, is much more compelling.

What does the real world say for weight loss?

I have known many people who genuinely felt DHEA helped them in many ways, including an improved feeling of well being, but none of them claimed to have lost any weight using it. In my personal experiences with people over the years, no one has lost measurable amounts of body fat from the use of DHEA.

Will Brink's Recommendation

It's well known that DHEA levels fall off as we age, and the research on health uses of DHEA justifies using small amounts to counter this age related drop off, or deficiencies from other causes.

As a muscle building supplement in young healthy athletes, DHEA is probably worthless, and high intakes may in fact be counterproductive to gaining muscle.

Positive effects of DHEA in older individuals is much clearer, however, with only 25-100 mg per day needed to positively effect bone mineral density, lean mass, and body fat levels in older men and women.

Why the difference between old and young people?

DHEA and DHEA–S levels are one of the best biological markers of aging known. DHEA levels rise slowly till they peak at around 30 years of age, and decline steadily after age 35, with levels reduced by 70-80% by age 75. This effect is one of the most consistent and predictable changes in aging people known so far.

Though the utility of DHEA in younger people with normal physiological levels of DHEA is debatable, the benefits clearly outweigh any small risks in people over 40 who have reduced DHEA levels.

Only blood tests will tell a person what their DHEA/DHEA–S levels are and where they are compared to others in their age group.

People interested in using DHEA as a general health benefiting supplement, should have blood tests done to determine their levels of DHEA/DHEA–S before using this supplement.

For general DHEA replacement, very small amounts are needed, like 25-50 mg a day for men and even less for women.

As a weight loss supplement, it's generally been a bust. Also, though fairly safe, it's not an innocuous substance. DHEA is a steroid hormone and weak androgen. Some women have noticed increases in facial hair growth from using large amounts of DHEA.

Other names and synonyms for DHEA

(3-beta)-3-Hydroxyandrost-5-en-17-one
(3beta)-3-Hydroxyandrost-5-en-17-one
3-beta-Hydroxy-5-androsten-17-one
3-Hydroxyandrost-5-en-17-one
3beta-Hydroxyandrost-5-en-17-one
4-08-00-00994 (Beilstein Handbook Reference)
5,6-Dehydroisoandrosterone
5,6-Dehydroisoandrostorone
5,6-Didehydroisoandrosterone
5-Dehydroepiandrosterone
17-Chetovis
17-Hormoforin
Andrestenol
Androst-5-en-17-one, 3-beta-hydroxy-
Androst-5-en-17-one, 3-hydroxy-, (3-beta)- (9CI)
Androst-5-en-17-one, 3-hydroxy-, (3beta)-
Androst-5-en-17-one, 3beta-hydroxy- (8CI)
Androstenolone
BRN 2058110
Caswell No. 051F
Dehydroepiandrosterone
Dehydroisoandrosterone
DHEA
Diandron
Diandrone
EPA Pesticide Chemical Code 126510
Epiandrosterone, 5-dehydro-
GL 701
Gynodian
NSC-9896
Prasterone
Prasteronum
Prestara
Psicosterone
Siscelar plus
trans-Dehydroandrosterone
UNII-459AG36T1B
Source: http://chemsub.online.fr/name/dehydroepiandrosterone.html

7–Keto–DHEA

What is it?

3–Acetyl–7–oxo–dehydroepiandrosterone
(7–keto–DHEA), as the name implies, is a
metabolite of DHEA.

What is it supposed to do?

The claim for 7–keto–DHEA is that it
possesses the benefits of DHEA without
any of the potential downsides, such as
possible effects on sex hormone levels. It's
supposed to be more biologically active
but lacks the ability to cause changes in
hormone levels.

Some research suggests 7–keto–DHEA
may be the active metabolite responsible
for many of the health benefits of DHEA.

What does the research say?

In-vitro (test tube) studies with 7–keto–DHEA appear to show it has no
effect on steroid hormones and does not convert to sex hormones such as
testosterone, estrogens, etc. Interestingly, 7–keto–DHEA may have a
more pronounced thermogenic effect (the process the body uses to
convert stored calories into energy) than DHEA.

A few animal studies and in-vitro studies have shown this. But, no
studies in people to date have looked specifically at the thermogenic
effect of 7–keto–DHEA vs. DHEA.

Some animal research has also shown improvements in memory and
other cognitive functions. 7–keto–DHEA may have positive effects on

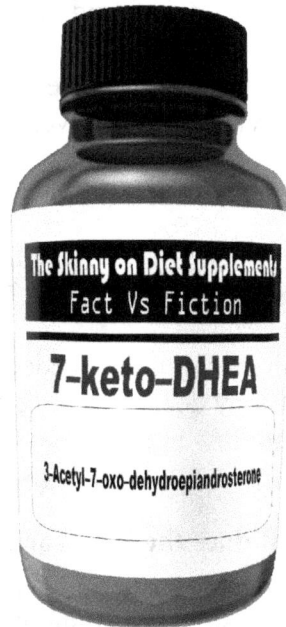

thyroid function. There has been one recent study that looked at weight loss in people. The study fed 30 overweight women (15 acted as a control group and received a placebo) 200 mg a day of 7–keto–DHEA for 8 weeks. The study found that the group getting the 7–keto–DHEA lost 1.8% of their bodyweight (a little over 6 lbs on average) vs. the placebo group who only lost 0.57% of their bodyweight.

The study also found that the group getting the 7–keto–DHEA had increases in the specific thyroid hormone T3 without significant changes in blood sugar, testosterone, estradiol (estrogen), liver, renal function tests, vital signs, or overall caloric intake over the eight week study.

The study conclusion was that

"... 200 mg of 7–Keto–DHEA per day yields a significant reduction in both body weight and body fat."

Further studies are needed to confirm this fat loss effect in people, but this study does make 7–keto–DHEA look like a potentially promising weight loss agent.

What does the real world say for weight loss?

7–keto–DHEA has gets mixed reviews from users. One of the major issues being, it's rarely if ever found alone and always found as part of a formula, making it very difficult to judge feedback from users.

Will Brink's Recommendation

On paper, 7–keto–DHEA looks promising. The single human study however, is a compelling one and appears to show 7–keto–DHEA as metabolic effects different from that of simple DHEA on weight loss. I consider 7–keto–DHEA one of those "might be worth a try" supplements at this time. It's not terribly expensive, appears safe, and may turn out to be something worthwhile as a weight loss nutrient. People interested in trying this supplement, can use 100-200 mg a day in divided doses.

DIGESTIVE ENZYMES

What are they?

Enzymes catalyze chemical reactions. As we all know, digesting our food involves many enzymes. There are various enzymes used in different digestive supplement formulas, some which are of animal origin and some of plant origin.

What are they supposed to do?

The breakdown of food starts in the mouth with chewing and the exposure to enzymes. In the stomach, food mixes with enzymes and other factors such as lipase, pepsin, intrinsic factor, and of course, hydrochloric acid (stomach acid).

The food moves on to the small intestine and then the large intestine. The small intestine is considered the major anatomical site of food digestion and nutrient absorption and is made up of sections such as the duodenum, jejunum, and the ileum.

Pancreatic enzymes (chymotrypsin, trypsin, etc.), bile salts, gastrin, cholecystokinin, and pepidases, are among the substances released here.

The large intestine is composed of the ascending colon, transverse colon, descending colon, and the sigmoid colon, which all play a part in absorbing the nutrients we eat.

Sounds complicated? It is.

Enzymes play an essential role in every step of the digestive process. The basic idea is that by adding specific enzymes in supplement form, it will help the body efficiently digest food and this will help with weight loss.

Companies market supplemental enzymes such as papain, amylase, lactase, lipase, bromelain, pancreatin, as well as others.

Enzyme therapy may have health benefits, especially for those with poor digestion or other issues relating to the digestive tract. Exactly how the enzymes are supposed to assist in weight loss in unclear.

What does the research have to say?

There are a few odd studies with animals that have found adding certain enzymes, such as pancreatin, reduced food intake and weight gain. One recent study fed broiler chickens large amounts of pancreatin and noted reductions in food intake and subsequent weight loss.

High amounts of pancreatin may have a mild anorectic (appetite suppressing) effect, but I doubt it would work in people or be particularly healthy either. However, there is very little modern research to go on regarding healthy people and weight loss with enzymes.

What does the real world say for weight loss?

I've never met a person who lost weight from taking enzymes as their only supplement.

Will Brink's Recommendation

Digestive enzymes have many potential health uses and are often prescribed for specific treatments in a variety of health problems, from simple digestion issues to pancreatitis and other pathologies. Some studies show the intake of certain enzymes, such as bromelain, may reduce inflammation. Other research suggests enzymes can positively affect immunity.

For weight loss specifically, enzymes don't appear to be any help. It's a wonder why so many diet books still recommend them.

It's impossible for me to give recommendations on how to take enzymes due to the fact there are so many types and formulas and each enzyme serves a different function. Enzyme formulas should pose no risk to healthy people however.

58

EPHEDRINE/CAFFEINE MIXTURES

What are they?

I am going to cover ephedrine and caffeine (EC) in one section as they are often found together in many "fat burner" type weight loss products. Ephedrine and caffeine are both mild to strong stimulants with many interesting properties.

Ephedrine can be derived from plants such as Ma Huang, Sida cordifolia, and others. It's also available in synthetic form, where it's used as an ingredient in over-the-counter (OTC) asthma medications.

Caffeine can be derived from kola nut, tea, guarana, and many other plant sources that contain it along with other compounds from the xanthine family.

What are they supposed to do?

EC products are called "thermogenic compounds" because they can increase thermogenesis (the production of heat) and affect metabolic rate.

Explaining everything ephedrine and caffeine do would take an entire book onto itself. It is my feeling most people purchased this book because they want short, concise, and easy to understand information regarding the many products on the market, not a long, drawn out and boring explanation of the science (or lack thereof) relating to each product.

So, in a nut shell, ephedrine is referred to as a beta–adrenergic agonist that works by mimicking the effects of the "fight or flight" hormones epinephrine and norepinephrine (i.e. adrenaline and noradrenaline).

The topic of beta–agonism can get complicated real fast, so we will leave it at that. The point is that beta–agonists such as ephedrine can have many positive effects relating to fat loss, such as increasing lipolysis (an increase in free fatty acids to be used as energy), increasing energy levels, preserving lean tissue (muscle) while dieting, and many other effects that greatly help with fat loss.

Caffeine is, of course, a chemical people are very familiar with and needs less explaining than ephedrine. Caffeine has effects similar to ephedrine but works through different mechanisms.

Ephedrine increases the release of norepinephrine, which modulates food intake and acts as a sympathomimetic agent to stimulate heart rate and blood pressure, and enhance thermogenesis.

Caffeine, on the other hand, is an adenosine antagonist and reduces the breakdown of norepinephrine within the synaptic junction.

Got all that? If not, don't worry. The point is simply that both compounds increase lipolysis, energy levels, etc., but use different pathways to do it.

One point that needs to be emphasized is that the actions of ephedrine and caffeine are not limited to lipolysis, but have other effects as well. Ephedrine also has anorectic (appetite suppressing) effects and helps increase energy levels before a workout. It can have a range of effects on the body, which is the reason why ephedra/ephedrine has been targeted by the FDA—unfairly, in my view.

In the discussion that follows, I'll do my best to explain the situation, and cut through the confusion that currently exists.

What does the research have to say?

The research on ephedrine and caffeine (EC) is clear and extensive regarding the effects on fat loss. Both caffeine and ephedrine alone have been found to be mildly helpful for weight loss, but together, there is clear synergism.

In other words, the effects of EC together are far more powerful than either compound alone.

Research published in the *American Journal of Clinical Nutrition* (55:246S–282, 1992*), International Journal of Obesity* (17[6]:343–347, 1993; S:73–78, 1993; 3:S73–77, 1993; 18:99–103, 1994), and the journal *Metabolism* (41[11]: 1233–1241, 1992; 41[7]:686–688, 1992; 40:323, 1990) as well as many others, have shown conclusively that the combination of E and C in the correct ratios and amounts is very effective for weight loss.

This research has been done on animals and confirmed repeatedly in human studies many times over the past decade.

The bottom line here is EC products work, and they work well for fat loss. A handful of clinical trials have shown that a C to E ratio of 10:1, that is ten times more caffeine than ephedrine, is an optimal ratio for this fat loss combination with minimal side effects.

The vast majority of studies have used 20 mg of ephedrine and 200 mg of caffeine three times a day for a total of 60 mg of E and 600 mg of C daily. Though a few studies suggest that lower doses may also be effective for weight loss, the vast majority have used the above doses.

Anecdotally, many report using half the standard recommended dose works well for fat loss with fewer side effects.

Those of you who are familiar with these products have usually known the above as the "ECA" combination which stands for ephedrine, caffeine, and aspirin. I have not covered this combination for a reason.

Though some studies suggest that the addition of aspirin may help with the fat loss effects of E and C, there has never been a head-to-head study done that showed the ECA combo was superior to the EC combo.

The vast majority of studies were in fact done on the EC combo. The value of including aspirin is questionable. There are even some theories that suggest adding aspirin may, in fact, hinder the fat loss effects of EC products.

In addition, taking aspirin on a daily basis in amounts needed for this stack, has potential side effects and health problems, such as burning a hole in your stomach.

Interestingly, EC research also shows lean tissue (muscle) is protected while on reduced calorie diets, which is another considerable plus for people using such products, especially athletes.

Another distinction of the EC products is that they appear to work on non-exercising people. There are very few supplements in the world that work on couch potatoes.

To be clear, I am not condoning sitting on your behind and using the ECA stack to lose weight, but it appears the ECA stack is effective for non-exercising (read: lazy) people.

In one recent study that examined the use of ECA with non-exercising people, subjects lost almost ten pounds of fat in six weeks from taking 20 mg of ephedrine, 200 mg of caffeine, and 325 mg of aspirin three times a day.

So what does this all tell us?

If the ECA combination works this well on couch po......err, sedentary people, imagine what it can do for people who get up off the couch and kick some butt in the gym!

What does the real world say for weight loss?

This is one of the few places where the research and the real world agree: EC products work for weight loss in the majority of people who use them.

Will Brink's Recommendation

Because EC, more specifically ephedrine, has been under such scrutiny regarding potential side effects, I am going to take extra time to address this issue. Between media sensationalism, the 2004 FDA ban and subsequent legal rulings, I can't blame people for being confused.

It's amazing to me that if a single study pops up on some new diet drug, no matter how obscure, the media leaps on it as if it were the cure for all weight problems. Yet when study after study on animals and people shows that a mixture of ephedrine and caffeine is a very effective and inexpensive method of fat loss, the media ignores it.

Why?

Beats me! They have been far more interested in attempting to show EC-based fat burners are inherently dangerous rather than showing them to be the safe and effective fat loss products they really are... and I base my conclusion on science and research rather than the anecdotal evidence favored by the "don't confuse us with the facts" media and FDA.

Do the people who want us to believe that ephedrine–based fat burners are inherently toxic ever bother to read the research on these products, or do they just ignore the studies? It's hard to tell.

Why don't the media ever give us both sides of the story and mention that studies to date using EC have come to the conclusion that these are safe products when used correctly?

Wish I knew!

Not only have there been multiple human studies showing weight loss with minimal side effects in healthy people, several studies have been done that specifically examined side effects.

One study called "**Ephedrine, Caffeine, and Aspirin: Safety and Efficacy for Treatment of Human Obesity**" concluded:

"In all studies, no significant changes in heart rate, blood pressure, blood glucose, insulin, and cholesterol levels, and differences in the frequency of side effects were found."

And where was this study conducted that the media never bothers to mention? A little out-of-the-way place called the Department of Medicine at the Harvard Medical School.

Another large randomized, placebo-controlled, double blind study with 180 subjects that ran for twenty four weeks called **"Safety and Efficacy of Long-Term Treatment with Ephedrine, Caffeine and Ephedrine/Caffeine Mixture"** concluded:

63

"The side effects are minor and transient and no withdrawal symptoms have been found."

This study—like the others—came to basically the same conclusion: that the side effects are minor (insomnia and tremors) and short lived. Not exactly what the media and the FDA would like us to believe regarding these products, no?

In healthy people who want to lose some weight, EC–based fat loss supplements have been proven repeatedly by human research to be both safe and effective. Are they completely harmless? Of course not, and I would never infer they were.

However, EC-based products are far from the killers the media and the FDA would have us believe. The FDA's decision to ban ephedra was overkill, and not grounded in either science or common sense.

Not only that, the FDA ban is inconsistent, and makes a confusing situation worse!

Due to the amazing logic of the "powers that be" ephedra for weight loss is banned, but due to the lobbying power of the pharmaceutical industry, ephedrine (the active principle in ephedra) is not banned for other uses and can be purchased in many drug stores or from online companies.

The more common brands are Bronkaid and Primatene, which are generally sold as asthma treatments. However, even these products are becoming more difficult for people to obtain.

Is it logical to ban the herbal form for dieters but allow ephedrine to be sold in any pharmacy? Hey, I don't make the laws…

If the above were not strange enough, the ban on ephedra was recently reversed…sort of.

Here's the scoop; A judge partially overturned the ban on ephedra by ruling the FDA action invalid. Without going into long detail over the court proceedings and boring you to tears, the decision only covers products that contain 10 mg or less of ephedrine alkaloids per daily dose—a much lower dosage than found to work in the studies and much lower than what is recommended in this book.

Separately, ephedra products are still unlawful in certain states that have banned the ingredient (e.g., California, Illinois and New York).

The decision nonetheless marks a significant victory for the dietary supplement industry. It does not, however, do much for those looking to take an EC product that actually has the dose required to cause fat loss!

All things considered, it's cheaper and easier—and also less confusing—to "roll your own" by going to the drug store and getting any one of the above listed ephedrine products if they're available. There are also some web sites dedicated to selling ephedrine that people report good experiences with, but I can't vouch for them.

Caffeine is sold in pill form under many names and is easy to find in any drug store. Presto, you have your EC stack in the doses and ratios this book recommends based on the research.

Who should not take this stuff

People who don't tolerate stimulants well, people with pre-existing medical conditions such as heart disease or any heart irregularities, high blood pressure, or prostate disease, pregnant women, and people taking MAO inhibitors are advised not to use EC in any form: herbal or "straight."

Taking more than the recommended dose

Another bad idea is taking far more EC than is needed. More isn't better, so stick to the recommended doses. It's a good idea to start with a lower dose of both (EC) and raise slowly over a few weeks until you reach those doses.

These particular warnings can be found on the side of many over-the-counter products used by millions of people every day, and they should not be ignored. A little common sense goes a long way here.

I generally advise people to use EC products for defined periods of time, with a specific off cycle. A good cycle for using EC products for maximum fat loss/minimum side effects is 8-14 weeks on and 2-6 weeks off.

If used as a pre-workout energy booster, I recommend using no more than 3-4 days per week.

Some additional considerations

When evaluating commercial EC products, take note of other compounds companies typically add to formulas such as cayenne pepper, tyrosine, and ginger—which they claim will enhance the fat loss/thermic effects of the EC combo. While they might help, there is no solid research to prove this.

There are also other stimulants included in "ephedra-free" fat burners that claim to be more thermogenic than EC with fewer side effects, such as norephedrine, theophylline, synephrine, and yohimbine (see section on yohimbine for more information), but none of them have been studied head-to-head in people to show they are superior to ephedrine for weight loss. Furthermore, they can have side effects of their own.

While combining these with EC might seem like a good idea (e.g., ephedrine and theophylline, etc.), I don't recommend it, as it could increase the potential for side effects above what is acceptable. If using any of the above stimulants or products in conjunction with EC products, I would recommend cutting back on the dose of EC to account for the additional effects.

Sources:

Nutraceutical Corporation v. Lester Crawford, **D.V.M., et al.**, Case No. 2:04CV409TC, U.S. District Court for the Central District of Utah

EVODIAMINE (EVODIA)

What is it?

Evodiamine is a bioactive alkaloid isolated from the dry, unripened fruits of Evodia rutaecarpa. Evodia rutaecarpa is used in traditional Chinese medicine to treat gastrointestinal disturbances and as an analgesic.

What is it supposed to do?

Evodiamine is alleged to raise core body temperature and accelerate fat burning.

What does the research say?

Evodia extracts slow the passage of food through the digestive tract by delaying gastric emptying and slowing intestinal transit (*Planta Med*. 1994 Aug;60(4):308–12.). This has been demonstrated only in rodent studies, but is consistent with its traditional use as an herbal remedy for diarrhea. It has anti-tumor activity and stimulates the release of acetylcholine, a neurotransmitter, in cell culture (test tube) studies.

It's also a vasodilator (*Pflugers Arch*. 2006 Jan 5;1–7); meaning it causes blood vessels to relax and expand.

There is a single study in rats that demonstrates evodiamine might have thermogenic and anti-obesity effects. When researchers added 0.02-0.03% Evodia extract to the rats' high-fat diet, the rats lost some fat and had lower blood lipids than controls. Fasting mice given 1-3 mg/kg evodiamine had increased heat production and heat loss (*Planta Med*. 2001 Oct;67(7):628–33.).

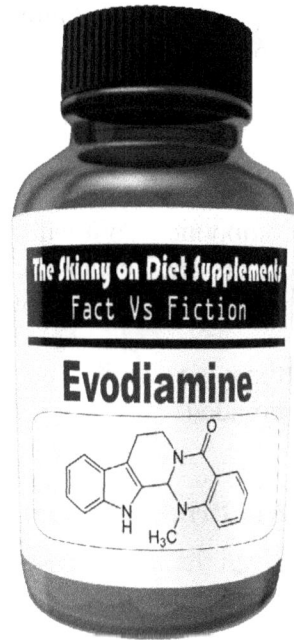

There are no human studies using either evodia extracts or evodiamine, but the animal studies cited above do at least look promising.

Too bad we are not mice…cheese and evodia extract anyone?

What does the real world say for weight loss?

Supplements containing Evodia extract/evodiamine are claimed to produce a warm, "shivering" response, which is probably due to its receptor binding and vasodilating effects. But user feedback is inconsistent-meaning, not everyone seems to experience this reaction.

Evodia extracts and/or evodiamine are sold in blends with other compounds, so it's difficult to evaluate what—if any—the fat loss effects are. Feedback on supplements containing them is mixed, and the results are inconsistent.

It may not work in humans, or it may be that an inadequate dose is provided.

Will Brink's Recommendation

Given the lack of research, I can't recommend evodia extracts or evodiamine for weight loss at this time. More research is clearly needed.

Don't waste your $$$ on this one. We don't even have a clue what the effective human dose is or if it's even effective in humans at all, much less the needed safety data!

FISH OIL

What is it?

As the name implies, we're talking about oils derived from fish. That's the easy part to remember. The "active" omega–3 lipids found in fish oil are EPA eicosapentaenoic acid (EPA) and docosahexaenoic acid (DHA). EPA and DHA are the "active" fatty acids that come preformed in fish, or can be formed in the human body from the essential fatty acid alpha linolenic acid (ALA).

Before you raise your hand to ask exactly what is an essential fatty acid; where does this ALA come from, and so on, that topic is fully covered in the section on flax oil, so don't overly concern yourself with it in this section. In this section, I examine fish oils (EPA/DHA) specifically and will fill in additional questions the reader may have in the following section on flax oil.

What is it supposed to do?

The term "omega–3 fatty acid" should ring a bell for you. Fish oils are well publicized sources of omega–3 fatty acids that have been shown to have many benefits.

The list of potential health benefits of fish oils is extensive, and beyond the scope of this section, but EPA and DHA are essential to brain and nervous system function development; and may help treat or reduce the risk of developing arthritis, high blood pressure, various cancers, and heart disease.

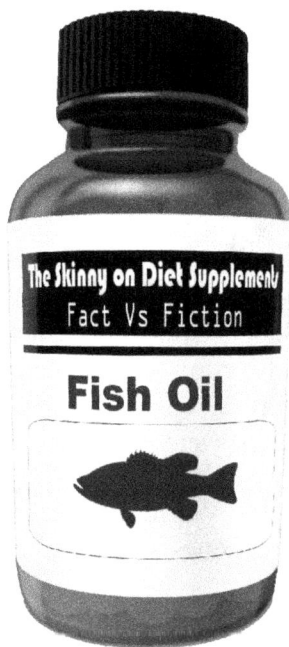

69

That's just the tip of the iceberg: the omega–3 fatty acids are anti–lipogenic (they block fat storage), anti-catabolic, anti-inflammatory, lipolytic (they increase fat burning!), improve insulin sensitivity, increase thermogenesis, and have a whole lot more positive effects on health that we don't have the space, time, or need to cover in this section.

Other studies find it may help with ADD, ADHD, depression, and autism! Yet other studies find fish oils may help relieve back and neck pain.

However, as fat loss is our focus here, so I will limit the discussion to that topic from here on.

Interestingly, research has found the omega–3 lipids control gene transcription. For the more technically adept readers, this means that omega–3 lipids play essential roles in the maintenance of energy balance and function as fuel partitioners. In this capacity, they direct glucose toward glycogen storage, and direct fatty acids away from triglyceride synthesis and assimilation and toward fatty acid oxidation.

Omega–3 lipids appear to have the unique ability to enhance thermogenesis and thereby reduce the efficiency of body fat deposition. EFAs exert their effects on lipid metabolism and thermogenesis by upregulating the transcription of the mitochondrial uncoupling protein–3, and inducing genes encoding proteins involved in fatty acid oxidation (e.g. carnitine palmitoyltransferase and acyl-CoA oxidase) while simultaneously down-regulating the transcription of genes encoding proteins involved in lipid synthesis (e.g. fatty acid synthase).

A lack of omega–3 lipids appears to be one of the dietary factors leading to the development of obesity and insulin resistance seen in Syndrome X (see section on chromium for more information of Syndrome X).

Finally, studies also find fish oil raises resting energy expenditure (REE) which should improve fat loss over time.

What does the research have to say?

Research has shown that adding omega–3 fatty acids to the diets of animals such as rats, mice and pigs results in fat loss. In animal studies, the effect has been quite consistent.

However, studies in humans with fish oils have suggested only moderate effects on fat loss or have been inconsistent.

In one study presented at the North American Association for Study of Obesity (NAASO) Annual Meeting, researchers gave fish oil supplements to 20 obese women (Body Mass Index above 40). The women were already on a very low calorie diet, with one group getting fish oil and another getting placebo. The group given the omega–3 supplements had a 20% greater weight loss than the group given placebo after only three weeks, with BMI reduced by as much as 15%.

That's one of the more impressive studies done with fish oils in people, and it may be an effect seen in a specific population of obese women severely lacking any omega–3 fats in their diets.

It should be noted however that not all studies in humans have had such dramatic results, possibly due to doses used, nutritional status of the study group, activity levels, and other variables. For example, in another study, researchers replaced 6 grams of fat with 6 g of fish oil (equal to 1.1 gram of DHA and 0.7 grams of EPA), in the diets of 6 men.

These men were allowed to eat their normal diets as they wished (ad libitum) for 12 weeks, while taking the fish oil supplements 3 times per day.

Their bodyweights did not change. However, their body compositions did change slightly, with a 2 lb loss of fat and an impressive 25% increase in beta–oxidation (fat burning!) which—over time, might have resulted in additional fat loss. A few lbs of fat loss (which didn't reach statistical significance) is not terribly impressive granted, but when you factor in the fact they were not on a diet or exercising, as well as the big increase in fat oxidation rates, it's a worthwhile study to note.

Regardless, the research has been generally favorable with fish oils in humans, though not as dramatic as the first study mentioned above.

What does the real world say for weight loss?

For the vast majority of people who have added fish oils to their diet, improved fat loss has been the result. How much fat loss seems to be fairly individual and depends on many factors and physiological variables such as diet, exercise, initial fatty acid status, dose, and body fat levels.

Fish oils are one of those supplements where the "real world" effects seem to consistently outpace what the research finds, as least where fat loss is concerned. Feedback for fish oils is almost universally positive.

Will Brink's Recommendation

Those who have read some of my articles on this will recall I had reservations about recommending fish oils. I wrote:

"In my view, there are reasons not to use the fish oils as the sole source of Omega–3 fats. They are far more susceptible to oxidation and rancidity. The production of fish oils for use as a supplement is not as well controlled as for flax seed oil and fish oils can contain toxins such as PCBs and other compounds. Fish oils do have their therapeutic uses however"

However, the quality of fish oil supplements across the spectrum of products has improved greatly in the past few years with the use of processing techniques such molecular distillation and others, which produces very high quality fish oil products. Of the major brands, such as The Life Extension® Foundation, Nordic Naturals®, and Carlson®, I would not worry much about that issue any more. I no longer have the above concerns for fish oil supplements, which is a good thing, considering how useful and healthy these products are.

On the issue of doses, it's not the amount of fish oil you take in, it's the amount if "active" lipids in the fish oil: EPA and DHA.

Obviously, 6 caps of fish oil containing 40% total active lipids is going to be a different dose than 6 capsules containing 30% active lipids, so you must read the labels for EPA and DHA content per capsule. In general, 30% active lipids—the combined amount of EPA and DHA in the product—is typical of most brands, but fish oil products with a higher percentage do exist, they just cost more but allow you to take fewer caps.

How much should you take?

Studies have used doses that are quite variable, so no exact dose is known in terms of optimal effects on fat loss, but 6-10 g/day (assuming 30% EPA + DHA) is a starting point. So, a 1000mg (1g) softgell cap of fish oil, would be approximately 180mg of EPA and 120mg of DHA, assuming the general rule of 30% total active lipids. Fish oil comes as 60/40 EPA to DHA.

I would recommend at least approximately 6g (which is 6 1000 mg caps) of fish oils giving you a total of 1800mg of active lipids per day assuming 30% of 6g is EPA and DHA, but you must read the labels for exact numbers.

Looking at specific brands for example:

Puritan's Pride®: Uses a 1200 mg capsule, each containing 360 mg total active lipids. You would need 5 capsules to equal 1800 mg total active lipids.

Life Extension® Foundation: They use a 1000 mg capsule that gives 600 mg total active lipids per cap, which means you would need 3 capsules to equal the recommended 1800 mg above.

Nordic Naturals®: They use a 1000 mg cap that gives a total of 275 mg of active lipids per capsule, so you will need 6-7 capsules per day

Carlson®: They use a 1000 mg cap that gives a total of 320 mg of active Omega–3 lipids, so you would need 5-6 capsules of this product.

Liquid vs. caps?

Several companies make liquid versions of their fish oil products, which can be both convenient and cost effective. There's no reason not to use the liquid versions if you don't mind the taste and you remember to read the labels for total active Omega–3 lipid content. For example, Carlson's makes a lemon favored liquid product that contains approximately the required amount of EPA and DHA in one teaspoon, so that's convenient and cost effective.

Higher doses

Can one use higher doses than listed above? Absolutely, and many do. Are higher doses more effective for fat loss? Unclear, but many feel higher doses are more effective, although the data is lacking there. If one uses higher doses, you will have to adjust calorie and fat intakes to account for much higher doses.

At the amount recommended in this section, the added calories are negligible, but at 10,000mg (10g) and higher, the additional fat and calorie content will need to be accounted for. That's not a negative per se, just something that does add additional complexity to your calorie and fat calculations during a fat loss phase.

Finally, although I'm sure I don't really need to say this at this point, fish oils get a thumbs up from me and I consider them an essential product during a diet.

FLAX OIL

What is it?

To understand flax oil you have to understand what essential fatty acids (EFAs) are and what they do. The definition of an essential nutrient is anything the body cannot synthesize itself and therefore must be obtained from the diet.

We need to eat an assortment of vitamins, minerals, approximately nine to eleven amino acids, and two fatty acids to stay alive and healthy.

The two essential fatty acids we need in our diets are Linoleic acid (LA) which is an omega–6 fatty acid and Alpha–Linolenic acid (LNA) which is an omega–3 fatty acid. The highest known source of the omega–3 fatty acid LNA is flax oil, which also contains a small amount of LA (flax oil has 4:1 ratio of LNA to LA).

Minimum requirements for essential fatty acids are 3-6% of daily calories for LA and 0.5-1% of daily calories for LNA.

What is it supposed to do?

As with most vitamins and minerals, it is virtually impossible to get optimal amounts of unprocessed essential fatty acids (especially the omega–3 fatty acids) from our heavily processed food supply.

The term "omega–3fatty acid" should ring a bell for you. Fish oils are well publicized omega–3 fatty acids that have been shown to have many benefits (see fish oil section for additional info). Although early research

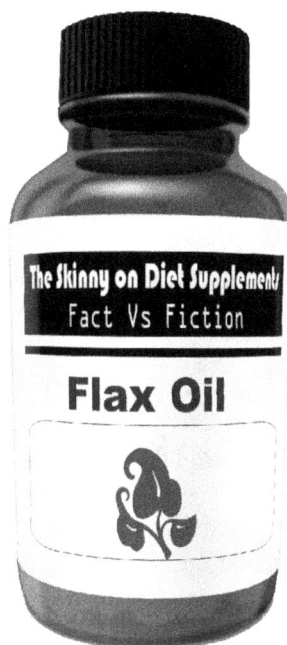

75

told us we need a bit more LA than LNA, in practice we find that a diet higher in LNA gets the best results for a reduction in body fat levels.

Americans tend to get their fats from saturated fats, rancid fats, and highly processed fats (which contain byproducts such as trans fatty acids), thus giving fats a bad name. EFAs are not to be avoided as a "bad fat" because all fats are not created equal. From a general health standpoint, EFAs are involved in literally thousands of bodily processes essential to our health and general well being. Immunity, aging, hormone production and hormone signaling, ...well, you get the point.

As one would expect, EFAs have been found to have many health uses including cholesterol reduction, cancer treatment and prevention and treating inflammatory conditions.

As mentioned in the fish oil section, and applicable here in the flax oil section:

"A lack of EFAs, in particular the omega–3 EFAs, appears to be one of the dietary factors leading to the development of obesity and insulin resistance seen in Syndrome X"

Of particular interest and importance, the body makes something called prostaglandins—in addition to other highly bioactive compounds such as thromboxanes, leukotrienes, and eicosanoids—from both of the essential fatty acids. Prostaglandins are highly active, short-lived hormone-like substances that regulate cellular activity on a moment to moment basis.

Prostaglandins are directly involved with regulating blood pressure, inflammatory responses, insulin sensitivity, immune responses, anabolic/catabolic processes, and hundreds of other functions known and yet unknown.

The long and the short of all this (without going into a long and boring biochemical explanation) is that omega–3 fatty acids are responsible for forming the anti-inflammatory prostaglandins, and omega–6 fatty acids are responsible for making many of the pro-inflammatory prostaglandins.

It's probably easy to see from just reading this section that the metabolism of EFAs is quite complicated. If you are interested in a solid, easy-to-read primer on the many functions of EFAs, flax and other oils, you should read *"Fats that Heal Fats that Kill"* by my good friend Dr. Udo Erasmus.

What does the research have to say?

The research that directly examines fat loss using flax oil is varied, compelling, and interesting, but not nearly as conclusive or extensive in humans as one would expect. Many of the benefits of listed in the fish oil section can be said of flax oil. However, there is also controversy there.

Most of the research over the years has in fact been done on the fish oils, and many people are already aware of such research. Flax oil and other high LNA oils have been more recently studied.

The human body can, in fact, make the "fish oils" EPA and DHA from the LNA found in flax oil, but some controversy still exists as to how efficiently it's converted which is why some recommend fish oils over flax.

What does appear clear is that conversion of LNA (from flax and other LNA rich oils) to the "active" lipids, EPA and DHA, can be altered by gender, diet, lack of co-factors for conversion (vitamin C, B6, B3, magnesium and zinc) various drugs, smoking, and perhaps, some inherent metabolic abilities for conversion between peoples and races.

Thus, as expected, studies have found a wide range of conversion of LNA to EPA—from a low of 0.2% to a high of 15%—and even lower for EPA to DHA. The large difference in these conversion rates may be due to differences in the studies themselves as well as factors already mentioned above.

What does the real world say for weight loss?

In the vast majority of people who have added flax oil to their diet, improved fat loss has been the result. How much fat loss seems to be fairly individual and depends on many factors and physiological variables such as diet, exercise, initial fatty acid status, and body fat levels.

Will Brink's Recommendation

Flax oil has been a particular interest of mine for years. As some people may already know, I was the first person to popularize the use of flax oil with bodybuilders and other athletes for fat loss. As I hope you can appreciate, I have attempted to distill a great deal of complicated information regarding the essential fatty acids and their effects on fat loss in this section, and I have of course left out a considerable amount of information. However, you should certainly get the gist of it.

General guidelines are to take 1-3 tablespoons of flax oil per day mixed in a protein drink, put over a salad with some vinegar, or taken straight from the bottle.

My recommendation is to use 1 tablespoon (14 g) per 75 lbs. of bodyweight for those who don't want to use fish oil.

Liquid vs. caps?

Don't bother with the capsules as it takes 12-14 capsules to equal one tablespoon, which becomes expensive and inconvenient.

A few important points to consider regarding flax oil

For one thing, flax oil, like all polyunsaturated oils, is very sensitive to heat, light, and oxygen. It should never be heated or cooked with and should be kept in the fridge after opening the bottle. Secondly, when a person increases their intake of such oils, they should also increase their intake of antioxidants such as vitamin C, E, selenium, and others. A good antioxidant complex is recommended.

Other oils

As previously mentioned, flax oil is particularly rich in omega–3 essential fatty acids (LNA) but is actually a poor source of the omega–6 fatty acid, LA. This makes flax oil too "omega–3 rich" and "omega–6 poor" for long term use.

78

Many writers on nutrition have made the mistake of telling people that flax oil is a good source of the essential fatty acids, which is not actually true. It is a good source of the omega–3 essential fatty acids but lacks adequate omega–6 EFAs.

There are two schools of thought on how to look at this problem as it relates to the essential fatty acids. The first says that most people already eat far too much omega–6 oils (which they do) and far too little omega–3 oils (also correct), and taking flax oil alone will bring you into balance.

The other camp believes flax oil is too rich in omega–3 essential fatty acids and taking it exclusively will lead to an omega–6 deficiency.

Where do I stand on this issue? I think both assumptions are correct depending on the population (or individual) you are looking at. What various companies have done is alter the ratio of omega–3 to omega–6 by mixing different oils together to get something closer to a 2:1 ratio of omega–3 to omega–6, as opposed to the 4:1 ratio of flax oil.

What this does is bring the ratio closer to what is optimal (and avoids any imbalances) while keeping it an omega–3 rich product that we find gets the best results. In addition, several companies have added other important and useful ingredients for health and fatty acid metabolism such as: lecithin, vitamin E, GLA, etc.

As you can see from the above discussion, not only do we need to get adequate amounts of both the essential fatty acids (LNA and LA), but we need to take them in the proper ratios with respect to one another. I have recently seen some of the companies that make these types of products, producing oils in a 1:1 ratio of LNA to LA, but I definitely prefer a product with more emphasis on the omega–3 essential fatty acids.

I have seen much better results in health, fat loss, and muscle gains, from an omega–3 rich product.

There are now all manner of mixed oil products out there such as Udo's Choice™, and oils with different ratios of EFAs, such as hemp, as well as others. There are also products such as Udo's + DHA, which uses an algal derived form of DHA, so it's close to a "best of both worlds" combination that would be excellent for vegetarians.

The inevitable comparison: fish oils vs. flax for fat loss

So you've read the fish oil section and now this section, and have the inevitable question "do I take flax or fish oils?" to lose fat, I recommend you use fish oils.

The reason is not because one is qualitatively superior to the other per se, but because fish oil is a much more concentrated source of the "active" preformed lipids EPA and DHA, which means far fewer fat calories coming from the fish oil. This gives you much more wiggle room with your fat calories when on low calorie intakes.

If using flax as the source of omega–3 lipids, you need considerably more of it to get the same amount of "active lipids" which makes is harder to fit other fats into your diet from the foods you eat and or from other sources, such as olive oil, etc. Thus, if following a diet to lose fat, which means you will be in a calorie deficit and need to be careful with your fat sources, the fish oil recommendation.

However, if not in a calorie deficit, then using flax or Udo's or some other blended oil product is fine. I use both. I will cut my fish oil dose in half, and add Udo's or flax oil into my diet if not attempting to lose fat, which means my calorie intake is higher and I have more room to play with fat calories.

So, when dieting, use fish oil, and get your other fats from naturally occurring sources from the foods you eat, small amounts of olive oil, etc. When not dieting/eating higher calories, you can use flax/Udo's or both (flax + fish, Udo's + fish, Hemp + fish, etc.), as it fits into your calorie requirements.

Flax, and other EFA-rich oils, get an unqualified thumbs up from me, but must be used intelligently, depending on total calorie intakes and goals.

FORSKOLIN

What is it?

Forskolin is extracted from the herb Coleus forskohlii, which grows in temperate areas such as India, Burma and Thailand. The herb is a member of the mint family and is commonly used as a traditional (Ayurvedic) medicine in India.

What is it supposed to do?

Forskolin may have various effects, but its major effect appears to be as an activator of adenylate cyclase. Adenylate cyclase is the enzyme involved in the production of cyclic adenosine monophosphate (cAMP), which is known as a "second messenger" in the cascade that ultimately leads to an increase in thermogenesis, lipolysis, and other metabolic effects that favor fat loss.

What does the research say?

Most of the studies with forskolin showing the effects on cAMP were done in-vitro (test tube) systems. In-vitro studies are interesting, but often have little bearing on results obtained with living systems (e.g., mice, rats, and humans).

Some studies using animals and humans do exist, although most of them are small and suffered serious methodological flaws, making them close to worthless. For example, one study often touted by sellers of forskolin was done with 6 people and was an open-field study, which means it was essentially uncontrolled. Ergo, it's a worthless study.

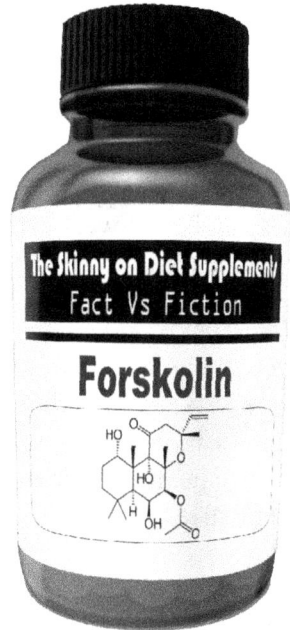

In general, the few studies done with human subjects are quite weak. More recent studies done under more controlled conditions using larger numbers of people have shown some promise, however.

A study published in the August 2005 Journal of Obesity Research entitled **"Body Composition and Hormonal Adaptations Associated with Forskolin Consumption in Overweight and Obese Men"** found a patented forskolin extract (see below) was moderately effective for fat loss.

This was a randomized, double-blind, placebo-controlled study of 30 overweight and obese men and ran for 12 weeks. Study participants were given either 250 mg of 10 percent forskolin extract twice daily or a placebo for 12 weeks and supposedly followed their normal diet and exercise routines.

The study found an average of a 9 lbs. (8.77 lbs.) increase in lean body mass, and approximately a 10 lbs. (9.96 lbs.) decrease in body fat vs. placebo—which had no statistically significant changes in lean body mass or body fat. The study found no statistically significant changes in various health parameters such as in blood pressure or other blood chemistries.

What does the real world say for weight loss?

In general, feedback from people using Coleus forskohlii extracts for weight loss has been lackluster. There maybe various reasons for that however (see below).

Will Brink's Recommendation

Up until recently, due to the lack of research and lackluster feedback, I would have put forskolin into the "not worth using" section of the ratings system in the book. Due to this aforementioned study I am going to put it into the "might be worth a try" category.

But clearly forskolin has not lived up to its in-vitro hype and promise.

One of the possible reasons the feedback has been so poor may simply be due to the lack of quality products on the market. Many products claiming to contain the active compounds in Coleus forskohlii were junk and contained little to no actual forskolin.

One company leading the way in terms of producing a standardized extract is the Sabinsa Corporation, which has a patented extract called ForsLean® (U.S. Patent #5,804,596 and European Patent #98,9075,379) which was the extract used in the study mentioned above.

For people interested in trying forskolin, I would recommend they find companies using this ForsLean® extract and use the dose the study found effective, which was 250 mg of 10 percent forskolin extract twice daily. So far, forskolin appears to be quite safe.

Possible drug interactions to be aware of

Major Interaction Do not take this combination

Medications for high blood pressure (Calcium channel blockers) interacts with FORSKOLIN

Forskolin might decrease blood pressure. Taking forskolin with medication for high blood pressure might cause your blood pressure to go too low.

Some medications for high blood pressure include nifedipine (Adalat, Procardia), verapamil (Calan, Isoptin, Verelan), diltiazem (Cardizem), isradipine (DynaCirc), felodipine (Plendil), amlodipine (Norvasc), and others.

Medications that increase blood flow to the heart (Nitrates) interacts with FORSKOLIN

Forskolin increases blood flow. Taking forskolin with medications that increase blood flow to the heart might increase the chance of dizziness and lightheadedness.

Some of these medications that increase blood flow to the heart include nitroglycerin (Nitro-Bid, Nitro-Dur, Nitrostat) and isosorbide (Imdur, Isordil, Sorbitrate).

Moderate Interaction Be cautious with this combination

Medications that slow blood clotting (Anticoagulant / Antiplatelet drugs) interacts with FORSKOLIN

Forskolin might slow blood clotting. Taking forskolin along with medications that also slow clotting might increase the chances of bruising and bleeding.

Some medications that slow blood clotting include aspirin, clopidogrel (Plavix), diclofenac (Voltaren, Cataflam, others), ibuprofen (Advil, Motrin, others), naproxen (Anaprox, Naprosyn, others), dalteparin (Fragmin), enoxaparin (Lovenox), heparin, warfarin (Coumadin), and others.

Source: WebMD
http://www.webmd.com/vitamins-supplements/ingredientmono-1044-FORSKOLIN.aspx?activeIngredientId=1044&activeIngredientName=FORSKOLIN

GH RELEASING SUPPLEMENTS

What are they?

There is a long list of supplements being sold claiming to either be human growth hormone (HGH or GH) or cause the release of GH. The number of nutrients claiming to be able to increase HGH levels is long.

The major products in this category currently being marketed can be broken down into three major categories, however. There are:

- Homeopathic GH, which claims to contain actual HGH

- Growth hormone-promoting nutrients (e.g., certain amino acids, vitamins, etc.)

- Secretagogues, which are short peptides that supposedly cause the release of GH.

What are they supposed to do?

The role of GH in the human body is extensive and rather complicated with many effects still being elucidated. GH is known to play an essential role in the regulation of body fat levels, immunity, muscle mass, wound healing, bone mass, and literally thousands of other functions both known and yet unknown.

GH is a peptide 191 amino acids long with a molecular weight of approx. 20,000. It is produced by the anterior pituitary gland, located at the base of the brain. The bulk of the effect accomplished by GH is performed by a related hormone (Insulin-like Growth Factor-1 or IGF–1), which is released predominantly by the liver and, to some extent, by other tissues in response to GH levels.

However, some recent data suggests GH has effects separate from its relationship to IGF–1.

It is well established that GH levels steadily decline as we age and is partially responsible for the steady loss of muscle mass, loss of skin elasticity, immune dysfunction, and many other physical changes that take place in the aging human body.

But explaining in detail the many roles GH plays in the human body is beyond the scope of this book.

GH releasing nutrients claim to release GH and thus have the positive effects associated with GH.

What does the research have to say?

Research with GH has been both interesting and conflicting. However, the bulk of research with actual injections of GH is compelling. In populations who have reduced GH levels—such as the elderly—injections of GH have been shown to: increase skin thickness and elasticity, improve healing time and reduce infection rates after surgery, decrease body fat, increase muscle mass, increase bone density, improve cholesterol levels (by decreasing LDL cholesterol and increasing HDL cholesterol), and improve exercise capacity.

We will examine the three sections separately:

GH releasing nutrients

The number of nutrients found to possibly cause a release of GH are many, and include the amino acids arginine, leucine, ornithine, and glutamine; vitamins such as niacin, choline and pantothenic acid, and non-vitamin nutrients such as melatonin as well as many others.

Although there is a good deal of data showing many of these nutrients can cause a release of GH to some degree, not one study has demonstrated the same effects in humans or animals as is seen with actual injections of GH as outlined above.

Homeopathic GH

These products claim to contain actual GH in extremely minute quantities, which is the nature of homeopathic products. Believers in homeopathy insist that a compound (in this case GH) can be diluted down to virtually undetectable levels and still have biological effects.

Regarding GH, this idea is full of problems. For one, the amounts found in these products are of no biological significance, and even if directly injected at those levels, would have no effects on muscle mass or body fat levels.

Another major issue is the fact that GH is a very delicate molecule and will not survive the digestive process as the 191 amino acid length of GH will be chopped up by digestive enzymes. There is no solid data showing any of these products effects muscle mass or body fat.

Secretagogues

A secretagogue is generally made up of short amino acid peptides 6-11 amino acids long, which may survive the digestive process and are orally absorbable. This has been an intensive area of research for pharmaceutical companies looking for a better way to increase GH levels instead of injections.

Some studies have shown these pharmaceutical compounds can stimulate the production of significant amounts of GH. For example, one secretagogue made by the huge pharmaceutical company Merck, is called NK677. Research looking at NK677 found it increased the size and frequency of the GH pulse during GH production.

Did this natural "pulse" of GH have an improved anabolic response over big single injections as studied in the previous research mentioned above? The answer appeared to be no, as there were no changes in muscle mass, strength or body fat in young weight lifters or older people who where given NK677.

To date, there is no data showing any of the "natural" secretagogues being sold on the supplement market alter body fat, muscle mass, or performance, much less the real pharmaceutical versions that are still being researched.

What does the real world say for weight loss?

The feedback on such products for increasing muscle mass or decreasing body fat has been almost universally negative.

Will Brink's Recommendation

There are many problems with this category of supplements.

For example, the age and GH status of the person appears to have a great deal to do with any GH being released, and many factors will dictate how much if any GH is does get released.

I have not listed doses for the above nutrients because they vary widely from nutrient to nutrient. But I will say is that some data also suggests that other counter-regulatory hormones such as the catabolic (muscle wasting) hormone cortisol may go up in response to such products.

None of the GH releasing products listed above have ever been shown to keep GH levels sustained and/or reach high enough levels—as injections of real GH have achieved—which appears necessary to see any real effects in body fat levels or muscle mass.

Also, in younger individuals with normal GH levels, even GH injections seem to be of little to no benefit.

The benefits of GH injections may be of real use in older populations who suffer from low GH levels. The truth is, GH levels go up and down all the time and can be altered by all sorts of things, from exercise, to standing in the cold, to hitting yourself on the head with a hammer…

So, the bottom line is?

Even if the current "GH releasing" products on the market do have some effects on GH (and I am not convinced they do), there is no reason to believe at this time they will effect muscle mass or body fat.

Sellers of such products make them look like the best thing since sliced bread by listing all the known effects of GH in the human body, then pretending their products have been proven to mimic those effects. The problem is they have not been shown to do this and probably never will.

Even much of the research using injections of real GH is often conflicting.

For example, one study looked at both young and old people given fairly large doses of GH and put on a weight lifting program. Both groups were given 40 mcg per kg of GH daily, which is a good sized dose.

As alluded to above about supplements that claim to raise GH, it's one thing to raise the level of some hormone but a totally different thing to show that a raise in that hormone is leading to more muscle mass or less body fat. **That is, who cares if the product raises some hormone if in the end it has no effect on muscle mass or body fat?!**

This research found that GH didn't increase protein synthesis or decrease protein breakdown (anti-catabolism) in the young guys lifting weights, even though their IGF–1 levels tripled. There were also no changes in strength between the GH group and the placebo group.

In the older group, the guys getting the GH did gain more fat-free mass (FFM) than the placebo group. However, the additional FFM turned out to be almost all water and not actual protein accumulation in the group getting the GH. Both groups showed similar strength increases.

So, in total, the amount of actual muscle gained by the older group getting GH was "nada" and it didn't do anything for their strength either.

Their conclusion was that large doses of GH combined with weight training has no additive effects over that of just weight training and IGF–1 levels went up without anabolic effect.

They did however feel that small multiple doses of GH would work better than one large whopping dose as this study used.

So much for GH being the "Holy Grail" of fat loss hormones!

This is not to say that GH does not play an important role in the body as a regulator of muscle growth and fat loss, but it is very clear that it is far more complicated than simply raising this hormone by injection or supplements.

Another important thing to know: chronically high GH levels are not by default a good thing and can come with side effects over time, such as insulin resistance, various neuropathies, and other problems.

In case you have not figured it out by now, I consider GH-releasing supplements to be perhaps the most over hyped supplements on the market for losing body fat and/or increasing muscle mass, especially in younger (under 40) people who eat well and workout.

For older individuals who have confirmed low GH levels, GH therapy by injections given by a medical doctor might be worth pursuing. As for safety, the GH releasing supplements appear safe enough.

GLUCOMANNAN

What is it?

Glucomannan (GM) is a highly purified, water-soluble dietary fiber that is derived from the konjac root (Amorphophallus konjac) also known as elephant yam.

What is it supposed to do?

GM is a very soluble and highly viscous dietary fiber that, like any fiber, adds bulk to the diet. Evidence suggests that GM exerts some of its beneficial effects by promoting satiety, and perhaps, the release of certain hormones involved in satiety (e.g., CCK, etc).

GM has an extraordinarily high water holding capacity, forming highly viscous solutions when dissolved in water. It has the highest molecular weight and viscosity of any known dietary fiber.

What that means in plain English is that GM absorbs a huge amount of water which causes it to expand, and that expansion leads to a feeling of fullness or satiety. Of course this is the effect seen with fiber in general and foods high in fiber, thus why higher fiber diets are recommended in general when trying to lose weight.

Like other forms of dietary fiber, GM is a "bulk-forming fiber" so it comes as no surprise that it makes for an effective laxative. As is the nature of fiber in the diet, GM may help with blood sugar regulation, reduce cholesterol levels and other blood carried lipids, and increase satiety (by increasing bulk in the stomach) which can lead to reduced calorie intakes.

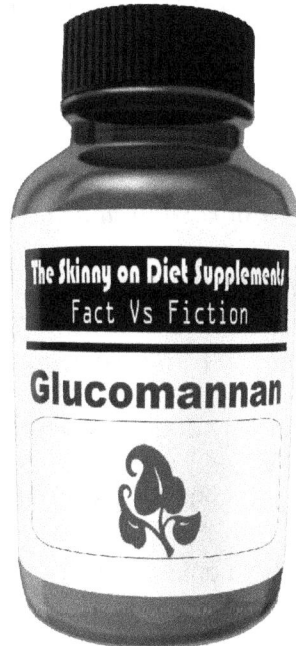

91

What does the research say?

Glucomannan may help weight loss by simply adding bulk (i.e., occupying space in the stomach), thus making a person feel full. Studies looking at GM for weight loss have generally been positive with a few exceptions.

A study done back in 1984 (*Int J Obes*. 1984;8(4):289–93.) found that subjects given 1g of GM an hour prior to meals, three times/day (for a total of 3 g), experienced a mean weight loss of 5.5 lbs. over the eight week study period.

The authors concluded:

"Results showed a significant mean weight loss (5.5 lbs.) using glucomannan over an eight-week period. Serum cholesterol and low-density lipoprotein cholesterol were significantly reduced (21.7 and 15.0 mg/dl respectively) in the glucomannan treated group. No adverse reactions to glucomannan were reported."

A study done in severely obese subjects also had positive findings with GM and weight loss, as well as other health related parameters (*Minerva Med*. 1992 Mar;83(3):135–9.).

They concluded:

"...due to the marked ability to satiate patients and the positive metabolic effects, glucomannan diet supplements have been found to be particularly efficacious and well tolerated even in the long-term treatment of severe obesity."

Several additional studies have found more or less similar results with a recent review (*Altern Ther Health Med*. 2005 Nov-Dec;11(6):30–4.) concluding:

"At doses of 2-4 g per day, GM was well-tolerated and resulted in significant weight loss in overweight and obese individuals."

All is not perfect however as a recent study (*J. Nutr*. 136: 384–389, 2006.) found no effects of 3 g per day of GM on weight loss above diet alone in another group.

What does the real world say for weight loss?

Feedback with GM has been limited, so no useful feedback to report.

Will Brink's Recommendation

Studies looking at weight loss specifically with GM have used 1-3 g prior to meals. It seems prudent users would want to start at a low dose (say 500 mg) and work their way up. Although the studies have found GM to be generally well tolerated, most people aren't used to high amounts of fiber in their diet and problems such as abdominal pain and bloating (intestinal gas) have been reported.

It's recommended that 10 ounces of water be taken with each dose of GM prior to meals.

I have mixed feelings about recommending GM as a weight loss supplement. Although studies have generally been positive with minimal side effects, it's a supplement that attempts to correct a problem that can be corrected with food, namely the lack of fiber in most people's diets. Picking the right sources of carbohydrates that are high in fiber vs. taking a fiber supplement makes far more sense.

GM supplies no nutrients other than fiber whereas most foods high in fiber supply many nutrients such as vitamins, minerals, various phytonutrients, etc.

Eating the low GI, high fiber foods will lead to essentially the same results, which is an improvement in blood lipids, a feeling of satiety with meals and improvements in blood sugar regulation.

Because most studies find GM effective for weight loss and no serious side effects have been reported, GM will be added to the "might be worth a try" list, but the reservations I have mentioned above should be noted by readers.

Possible drug interactions to be aware of

Moderate Interaction Be cautious with this combination

Medications for diabetes (Antidiabetes drugs) interacts with GLUCOMANNAN

Glucomannan can decrease blood sugar in people with type 2 diabetes. Diabetes medications are also used to lower blood sugar. Taking glucomannan along with diabetes medications might cause your blood sugar to go too low. Monitor your blood sugar closely. The dose of your diabetes medication might need to be changed.

Some medications used for diabetes include glimepiride (Amaryl), glyburide (DiaBeta, Glynase PresTab, Micronase), insulin, pioglitazone (Actos), rosiglitazone (Avandia), chlorpropamide (Diabinese), glipizide (Glucotrol), tolbutamide (Orinase), and others.

Medications taken by mouth (Oral drugs) interacts with GLUCOMANNAN

Glucomannan absorbs substances in the stomach and intestines. Taking glucomannan along with medications taken by mouth can decrease how much medicine your body absorbs, and decrease the effectiveness of your medication. To prevent this interaction, take glucomannan at least one hour after medications you take by mouth.

Source: WebMD
http://www.webmd.com/vitamins-supplements/ingredientmono-205-GLUCOMANNAN.aspx?activeIngredientId=205&activeIngredientName=GLUCOMANNAN

GLYCOMACROPEPTIDES (GMP)

What is it?

Glycomacropeptide (GMP) is a protein sub-fraction found in some whey protein supplements. Whey proteins are derived from cow's milk and contain many sub-fraction proteins and peptides, including GMP.

When we talk about whey protein we are actually referring to a complex mixture made up of many smaller protein and peptide sub-fractions such as: beta–lactoglobulin, alpha–lactalbumin, immunoglobulins (IgGs), glycomacropeptides, bovine serum albumin (BSA), along with minor amounts of lactoperoxidases, lysozyme, and lactoferrin.

Each of the sub-fractions found in whey has its own unique biological properties.

Whey protein appears to be a powerful natural food with a host of positive effects on human health, such as improved immunity.

I will go more in depth about whey in the following section.

What is it supposed to do?

GMP may be able to help people trying to lose weight by stimulating the release of a hormone called cholecystokinin (CCK). CCK has many functions in the human body. CCK plays an essential role relating to

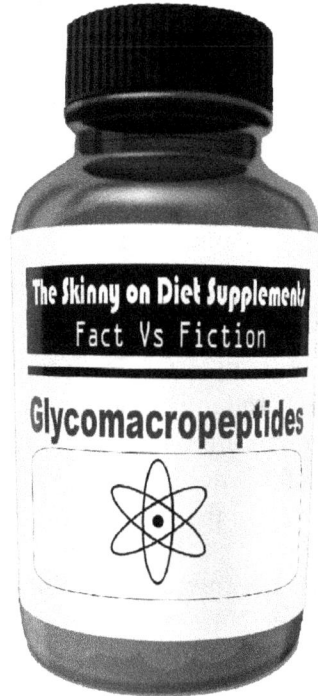

gastrointestinal function, including the regulation of food intake in animals and (hopefully) humans.

In addition to being a regulator of food intake, CCK stimulates gallbladder contraction, stimulates bowel motility, regulates gastric emptying, and stimulates the release of enzymes from the pancreas. CCK also has effects on the central nervous system.

In particular, CCK is often referred to as a "satiety hormone," meaning it is a hormone that tells the brain when a person has eaten enough food. This means that CCK is considered to function as an important regulator of satiety and food intake.

What does the research say?

In animals, CCK is directly related to food intake. Increases in CCK will cause reductions in food intake and consequently weight loss in many animals studied, such as mice, rats, and dogs. Interestingly, newborn infants who are breast fed have much higher levels of CCK and take in less food than formula fed infants.

Another interesting tidbit is that one of the ways nicotine may exert its anorectic (appetite suppressing) effects is by raising CCK.

In rats exposed to nicotine, CCK levels are much higher and food intake much lower, resulting in weight loss. In humans, the exact relationship of CCK to food intake and weight loss is not as clear (so what else is new?) though CCK is clearly related on some level to food consumption. In the past few decades, the mechanisms of what signal tells people to stop eating (i.e., the satiating effect of food that terminates a meal) have been clinically investigated in animals and humans.

The research revealed that peptides such as cholecystokinin (CCK), pancreatic glucagon, and bombesin are released by ingested food in the gastrointestinal tract and are related to food intake. The release of these gut based peptides appears to decrease meal size in a dose related manner without toxicity.

Perhaps more importantly to people, the stimulation of these peptides appears to decrease meal size without decreasing the reported pleasure or satisfaction of the meal.

Research into the use of these peptides may find them to be a new class of appetite suppressing agents, though more human research is needed. Recent studies in humans were not promising. There's limited, though interesting research showing GMP from whey increases CCK.

A clinical study done by a Dr. Maubois from France found that the ingestion of whey by healthy volunteers resulted in a substantial elevation in CCK being released. What he did not check, however, was if this large increase in CCK resulted in less food being consumed or if any weight loss occurred.

Although there's been some very compelling animal research that suggest GMP very promising, the effect was not supported by recent human research that failed to find GMP—or whey without GMP— reduced food intake or improved satiety.

Currently, the research is conflicting, so that's the best that can be said at this time.

What does the real world say for weight loss?

This is not one of those things where people can say "my CCK went up, and I ate less and lost weight from using whey supplements containing GMP."

However, it has been observed that the use of whey protein supplements during a diet seems to make dieting easier for most people.

Many athletes, especially many heavily into fitness, rely heavily on whey based supplements when dieting. Whether or not this is related in some small part to a release of CCK by GMP is of course unknown, and many other factors could be related to this positive feedback regarding whey as whey is a complex protein with many sub fractions and various constituents that may impact different pathways and mechanisms involved in appetite and or metabolism.

97

Will Brink's Recommendation

If GMP in whey is ultimately found to be great for weight loss, then the people using whey will be ahead of the game. If not, they will still be using a very high quality source of protein with a long list of potential health benefits.

However, specific to GMP and having direct effects on weight loss, via reduced food intake and increased satiety, recent human research did not support that affect (The influence of whey protein and glycomacropeptide on satiety in adult humans. *Physiol. Behav.* 2009 Jan 8;96(1):162-8.).

A few important points however: GMP in whey can range from 0-25%, depending on how the whey is produced. For example, ion-exchange whey proteins (a popular type of whey used by athletes) contain virtually no GMP. Whey proteins are very persnickety about how they are processed, and many of the sub-fractions are easily lost due to certain processing methods employed.

I recommend well made whey using processes that preserve the sub-fraction ratios naturally found in the whey. Cross-flow microfiltration (CFM™) is one process that does a great job of this.

If you're interested in knowing more about the issue of whey processing and the preservation of peptides found in whey (i.e. GMP, etc.) check out my article on Brinkzone.com for more information as the topic is too complicated and detailed to cover here.

People wishing to use whey as a possible adjunct to weight loss can try one scoop 30-40 minutes prior to meals one to three times per day. Athletes often use more, up to six or more scoops per day (most scoops are a 20 g serving).

There are no known side effects of using whey proteins, though individuals with milk allergies should try a small amount first and consult their doctor.

Although CCK is linked to the control of human food intake, people should understand it's a very complicated system in human beings— much more so than in mice and rats.

There is a great deal of research going on concerning drugs to reduce appetite, and some should be hitting the market in the not-too-distant future. One such drug is called C75.

Originally, C75 was being tested as a cancer drug when it was found to have a remarkable effect on weight loss and food intake. C75 appears to be using a major pathway in the brain the body uses to signal when it has eaten enough food. In one day, C75 reduced food intake by more than 90% in mice!

The hypothalamus appears to be the part of the brain (known as the limbic system) that is involved in the regulation of hunger and eating. By mapping blood flow in the brain, scientists have found it takes approximately 10 minutes for the human brain to receive the signal that the stomach is full after a meal.

Amazingly, one recent study found this system works differently in thin people vs. overweight people. That is, the brain's response to food is significantly different in thin people vs. fat people.

Although humans and mice are quite different, we humans are known to have a similar mechanism in the brain controlling hunger and C75 seems to work in the appetite center of the brain.

C75 may work by altering levels of hormones such as leptin or neuropeptide Y, both of which are known to control appetite and hunger in man and animals. This is only the tip of the iceberg regarding new research and drugs that get to the heart of the obesity problem, especially in affluent countries such as the US.

Controlling the signals of hunger and appetite (no they are not the same thing) is the key to weight loss, and future drugs will work by manipulating CCK, leptin, neuropeptide Y, to name the major players. The use of GMP may be a major step in that direction.

"But wait a second! GMP is in whey, what about that?" you ask. OK...

WHEY PROTEIN

This particular section does get a bit heavy in the technical and scientific areas, so apologies ahead! However, it would serve you well to at least attempt to wade through this section.

Whey has a wide variety of potential benefits, such as effects on immunity, fight cancer, and improve glutathione levels are well documented in animal studies and supported by additional human studies.

Additional research suggests possible medical uses for whey that are quite unexpected and different from whey's traditional role as an immune booster and anti-cancer functional food.

For example, whey may be able to reduce stress, lower cortisol, increase brain serotonin levels, improve liver function in those suffering from certain forms of hepatitis, reduce blood pressure, as well as other amazing recent discoveries, such as whey's possible effects on weight loss, which is the real focus of this book.

What is it?

As outlined in the GMP section, whey is a milk-based ingredient made up of protein, lactose, fat and minerals. Protein is the best known component of whey and is made up of many smaller protein sub-fractions such as: Beta–lactoglobulin, alpha–lactalbumin, immunoglobulins (IgGs), glycomacropeptides (GMP), bovine serum albumin (BSA) and minor peptides such as lactoperoxidases, lysozyme and lactoferrin.

Each of the sub-fractions found in whey has its own unique biological properties. Modern filtering technology has improved dramatically in the past decade, allowing companies to separate some of the highly bioactive peptides—such as lactoferrin and lactoperoxidase—from whey.

Some of these sub-fractions are only found in very minute amounts in cow's milk; normally at less than one percent (e.g., lactoferrin, lactoperoxidase, etc.)

The medicinal properties of whey have been known for centuries. For example, an expression from Florence, Italy. Circa 1650, was *"Chi vuol viver sano e lesto beve scotta e cena presto"* which translates into English as "If you want to live a healthy and active life, drink whey and dine early."

Another expression from Italy regarding the benefits of whey (circa 1777) was *"Allevato con la scotta il dottore e in bancarotta."* Which translates into English "If everyone were raised on whey, doctors would be bankrupt."

What is it supposed to do?

Whey protein is an extremely high quality source of essential amino acids that are easily digested and absorbed. But beyond its value as a source of dietary protein, it possesses a variety of potential health and possible weight loss benefits.

Is whey a weight loss functional food?

A few years ago, I might have said no. Now I am not so sure. Although there was a smattering of studies suggesting whey had certain properties that might assist with weight loss, a number of recent studies appear to further support the use of whey as a possible weight loss supplement.

Most interesting—at least to nerds like me—the effect appears to be not by a single mechanism, but several. I will briefly explore a few possible pathways by which whey may assist the dieter.

"I'm hungry!"

Human hunger and appetite are regulated by a phenomenally complicated set of overlapping feedback networks, involving a long list of hormones, psychological factors as well as physiological factors, all of which are still being elucidated. It's a very intensive area of research

102

right now, with various pharmaceutical companies looking for that "magic bullet" weight loss breakthrough they can bring to market.

One hormone getting attention by researchers looking for possible solutions to obesity is cholecystokinin (CCK). Several decades ago, researchers found CCK largely responsible for the feeling of fullness or satiety experienced after a meal and partially controls appetite, at least in the short term.

Cholecystokinin (CCK) is a small peptide with multiple functions in both the central nervous system and the periphery (via CCK–B and CCK–A receptors respectively). Along with other hormones, such as pancreatic glucagon, bombesin, glucagon-like peptide–1, amide (GLP–1), oxyntomodulin, peptide YY (PYY) and pancreatic polypeptide (PP)., CCK is released by ingested food from the gastrointestinal tract and mediates satiety after meals.

Such a list would not be complete without at least making mention of what many researchers consider the "master hormones" in this milieu, which is insulin and leptin. If that's not confusing enough, release of these hormones depends on the concentration and composition of the nutrients ingested. That is, the type of nutrients (i.e., fat, protein, and carbohydrates) eaten, the amount of each eaten, and composition of the meal, all effect which hormones are released and in what amounts.

Needless to say, it's a topic that gets real complicated real fast and the exact roles of all the variables is far from fully understood at this time, though huge strides have been made recently.

What does the research say?

This (finally!) brings us to whey proteins effect on food intake. Whey may have some unique effects on food intake via its effects on CCK and other pathways. Many studies have shown that protein is the most satiating macro-nutrient. However, it also appears all proteins may not be created equal in this respect.

For example, two studies using human volunteers compared whey vs. casein (another milk based protein) on appetite, CCK, and other hormones. The first study found that energy intake from a buffet meal ad libitum was significantly less 90 minutes after a liquid meal containing whey, compared with an equivalent amount of casein given 90 minutes before the volunteers were allowed to eat all they wanted (ad libitum) at the buffet.

In the second study, the same whey preload led to a plasma CCK increase of 60 % (in addition to large increases in glucagon-like peptide [GLP]-1 and glucose-dependent insulinotropic polypeptide) following the whey preload compared with the casein.

Translated, taking whey before people were allowed to eat all they wanted (ad libitum) at a buffet showed a decrease in the amount of calories they ate as well as substantial increases in CCK compared to casein. Subjectively, it was found there was greater satiety followed the whey meal also.

The researchers concluded:

"These results implicate post-absorptive increases in plasma amino acids together with both CCK and GLP-1 as potential mediators of the increased satiety response to whey and emphasize the importance of considering the impact of protein type on the appetite response to a mixed meal."

Several animal studies also find whey appears to have a pronounced effect on CCK and or satiety over other protein sources. But it should be noted however that not all studies have found the effect of whey vs. other protein sources on food intake.

It should also be noted that although studies find protein to be the most satiating of the macro-nutrients, certain protein sources (e.g. egg whites) may actually increase appetite, so protein sources appear worth considering when looking to maximize weight loss and suppress appetite.

How whey achieves this effect is not fully understood, but research suggests it's due to whey's high glycomacropeptide and alpha-lactalbumin content, as well as its high solubility compared to other proteins, and perhaps it's high percentage of branch chain amino acids (BCAA's).

Whey's effects on body fat, insulin sensitivity, and fat burning

So we have some studies suggesting whey may have some unique effects on hormones involved in satiety and or may reduce energy (calorie) intake of subsequent meals, but do we have studies showing direct effects of whey vs. other proteins on weight loss?

In animals at least, whey has looked like a promising supplement for weight loss.

Although higher protein diets have been found to improve insulin sensitivity, and may be superior for weight loss (with some debate!) then higher carbohydrate lower protein diets, it's unclear if all proteins have the same effects.

One study compared whey to beef and found whey reduced body weight and tissue lipid levels and increased insulin sensitivity compared to red meat.

Rats were fed a high-fat diet for nine weeks, then switched to a diet containing either whey or beef for an additional six weeks. As has generally been found in other studies, the move to a high dietary protein reduced energy intake (due to the known satiating effects of protein compared to carbs or fat), as well as reductions in visceral and subcutaneous body fat.

However, for the rats getting the whey, there was a 40% reduction in plasma insulin concentrations and increased insulin sensitivity compared to the red meat. Not surprisingly, the researchers concluded:

"These findings support the conclusions that a high-protein diet reduces energy intake and adiposity and that whey protein is more effective than red meat in reducing body weight gain and increasing insulin sensitivity."

Other studies suggest taking whey before a workout is superior for preserving/gaining lean body mass (LBM) and maintaining fat burning (beta oxidation) during exercise over other foods taken prior to a workout. The study called "**A preexercise lactalbumin-enriched whey**

105

protein meal preserves lipid oxidation and decreases adiposity in rats" (*Am J Physiol Endocrinol Metab* 283: E565–E572, 2002.) came to some very interesting conclusions.

One thing that's been known a long time is the composition of the pre-exercise meal will affect substrate utilization during exercise, and thus might affect long-term changes in body weight and composition.

So depending on what you eat before you workout can dictate what you use for energy (i.e. carbs, fats, and or proteins), which alters what you burn (oxidize) for energy.

The researchers took groups of rats and made the poor buggers exercise two hours daily for over five weeks (talk about over training!), either in the fasted state or one hour after they ingested a meal enriched with a simple sugar (glucose), whole milk protein or whey protein.

The results were quite telling. Compared with fasting (no food), the glucose meal increased glucose oxidation and decreased lipid oxidation during and after exercise. Translated, they burned sugar over body fat for their energy source.

In contrast, the whole milk protein and whey meals preserved lipid oxidation and increased protein oxidation; meaning, fat burning was maintained and they also used protein as a fuel source.

Not surprisingly, the whey meal increased protein oxidation more than the whole milk protein meal, most likely due to the fact that whey is considered a "fast" protein that is absorbed rapidly due to it's high solubility.

As one would expect, by the end of the five weeks, body weight was greater in the glucose, whole milk protein and whey fed rats than in the fasted ones. No shock there.

But here is where it really gets interesting; in the group getting the glucose or the whole milk protein, the increase in weight was from body fat, but in the whey fed group, the increase in weight was from an increase in muscle mass and a decrease in body fat!

Only the rats getting the whey before their workout increased muscle mass and decreased their body fat. The researchers theorized this was due to whey's ability to rapidly deliver amino acids during exercise.

Is this the next big find in sports nutrition or those simply looking to preserve muscle mass loss due to aging?

Hard to say at this time being it was done in rats, but if it turns out to be true in humans (and there is no reason people can't try it now) it would indeed be a breakthrough in the quest to add muscle and lose fat.

Effects on serotonin, blood sugar regulation, and more!

Although the above would probably be the major mechanisms by which whey could help the dieter, there are several secondary effects of whey that may assist in weight loss. For example, whey's effects on serotonin levels.

Serotonin is probably the most studied neurotransmitter since it has been found to be involved in a wide range of psychological and biological functions. Serotonin (also called 5-hydroxytryptamine or 5-HT) is involved with mood, anxiety, and appetite.

Elevated levels of serotonin can cause relaxation and reduced anxiety. Low serotonin levels are associated with low mood, increased anxiety (hence the current popularity of the SSRI drugs such as Prozac and others), and poor appetite control.

This is an extremely abbreviated description of all the functions serotonin performs in the human body—many of which have yet to be fully elucidated—but a full explanation is beyond the scope of this book.

Needless to say, Increased brain serotonin levels are associated with an improved ability of people to cope with stress, whereas a decline in serotonin activity is associated with depression and anxiety. Elevated levels of serotonin in the body often result in the relief of depression, as well as substantial reduction in pain sensitivity, anxiety and stress.

It has also been theorized that a diet-induced increase in tryptophan will increase brain serotonin levels, while a diet designed for weight loss (e.g., a diet that reduces calories) may lead to a reduction of brain serotonin levels due to reduced substrate for production and a reduction in carbohydrates.

Many people on a reduced calorie intake in an attempt to lose weight find they are often ill tempered and more anxious. Reductions in serotonin may be partially to blame here.

One recent study (**"The bovine protein alpha-lactalbumin increases the plasma ratio of tryptophan to the other large neutral amino acids, and in vulnerable subjects raises brain serotonin activity, reduces cortisol concentration, and improves mood under stress"** *Am J Clin Nutr* 2000 Jun;71(6):1536-1544) examined whether alpha-lactalbumin—a major sub-fraction found in whey which has an especially high tryptophan content—would increase plasma Tryptophan levels as well reduce depression and cortisol concentrations in subjects under acute stress considered to be vulnerable to stress.

The researchers examined twenty-nine "highly stress-vulnerable subjects" and 29 "relatively stress-invulnerable" subjects using a double blind, placebo-controlled study design.

The study participants were exposed to experimental stress after eating a diet enriched with either alpha-lactalbumin (found in whey) or sodium-caseinate, another milk based protein.

The researchers looked at:

- Diet-induced changes in the plasma Tryptophan and its ratio to other large neutral amino acids.
- Prolactin levels.
- Changes in mood and pulse rate.
- Cortisol levels (which were assessed before and after the stressor).

108

Amazingly, the ratio of plasma Tryptophan to the other amino acids tested was 48% higher after the alpha-lactalbumin diet than after the casein diet! This was accompanied by a decrease in cortisol levels and higher prolactin concentration.

Perhaps most important and relevant to the average person reading this is that they found "reduced depressive feelings" when test subjects were put under stress.

They concluded:

"Consumption of a dietary protein enriched in tryptophan increased the plasma Trp-LNAA ratio and, in stress-vulnerable subjects, improved coping ability, probably through alterations in brain serotonin."

This effect was not seen in the sodium-caseinate group. If other studies can confirm these findings, whey may turn out to be yet another safe and effective supplement in the battle against depression and stress, as well as reduced serotonin levels due to dieting.

Although there is a long list of hormones involved in appetite regulation, some of which have been mentioned above, serotonin appears to be a key player in the game.

In general, experiments find increased serotonin availability or activity = reduced food consumption and decreased serotonin = increase food consumption.

If whey can selectively increase serotonin levels above that of other proteins, it could be very helpful to the dieter.

Other possible advantages whey may confer to the dieter is improved blood sugar regulation which is yet another key area in controlling appetite and metabolism.

Finally, calcium from dairy products has been found to be associated with a reduction in bodyweight and fat mass. Calcium is thought to influence energy metabolism as intracellular calcium regulates fat cell (adipocyte) lipid metabolism as well as triglyceride storage.

It's been demonstrated in several studies the superiority of dairy versus non-dairy sources of calcium for improving body composition, and the whey fraction of dairy maybe the key.

The mechanism responsible for increased fat loss found with dairy-based calcium versus nondairy calcium has not is not fully understood but researchers looking at the issue theorized:

"...dairy sources of calcium markedly attenuate weight and fat gain and accelerate fat loss to a greater degree than do supplemental sources of calcium. This augmented effect of dairy products relative to supplemental calcium is likely due to additional bioactive compounds, including the angiotensin-converting enzyme inhibitors and the rich concentration of branched-chain amino acids in whey, which act synergistically with calcium to attenuate adiposity."

It appears components in whey—some of which have been mentioned above—are thought to act synergistically with calcium to improve body composition.

Will Brink's Recommendation

Whey protein is one of my personal interests and I have written as much, or more, on this topic than anyone. Whey is known to have so many potential health benefits not only to athletes and dieters, but everyone else, however, so that the addition of a few scoops of whey to any weight loss plan is a no-brainer in my book.

Taken in isolation, none of these studies are so compelling that people should run out and use whey as some form of weight loss nirvana.

However, taken as a total picture, the bulk of the research seems to conclude that whey may in fact have some unique effects for weight loss and should be of great use to the dieter. More studies are clearly needed however.

So what is the practical application of all this information and how does the dieter put it to good use?

Being the appetite suppressing effects of whey appear to last approximately 2-3 hours, it would seem best to stagger the intake throughout the day. For example, breakfast might be 1-2 scoops of whey and a bowl of oatmeal, and perhaps a few scoops of whey taken between lunch and dinner.

Sources:

Bowen J, Noakes M, Clifton P, Jenkins A, Batterham M. Acute effect of dietary proteins on appetite, energy intake and glycemic response in overweight men. *Asia Pac J Clin Nutr.* 2004;13(Suppl):S64.

Hall WL, Millward DJ, Long SJ, Morgan LM. Casein and whey exert different effects on plasma amino acid profiles, gastrointestinal hormone secretion and appetite. *Br J Nutr.* 2003 Feb;89(2):239-48.

Damien P. Belobrajdic, Graeme H. McIntosh, and Julie A. Owens. A High-Whey-Protein Diet Reduces Body Weight Gain and Alters Insulin Sensitivity Relative to Red Meat in Wistar Rats. J. Nutr. 134:1454-1458, June 2004.

Frid AH, Nilsson M, Holst JJ, Bjorck IM. Effect of whey on blood glucose and insulin responses to composite breakfast and lunch meals in type 2 diabetic subjects. Am J Clin Nutr. 2005 Jul;82(1):69-75.

Anderson GH, Tecimer SN, Shah D, Zafar TA. Protein source, quantity, and time of consumption determine the effect of proteins on short-term food intake in young men. J Nutr. 2004 Nov;134(11):3011-5.

Zemel MB. Role of calcium and dairy products in energy partitioning and weight management. Am J Clin Nutr. 2004 May;79(5):907S-912S.

GREEN TEA EXTRACT

What is it?

Green tea has been used in China, India, and other eastern countries—both as a beverage and medicinally—for centuries. In the west, black tea is by far the more common tea, but green tea is making great strides as a beverage in the west.

Green tea is prepared by steaming the leaves then allowing the leaves to dry, while black tea has an added step in that it is allowed to ferment. Because green tea is not allowed to ferment, green tea contains many compounds that would other wise be lost during the fermentation process. Both forms of tea contain caffeine.

In recent years, companies have been offering green tea extracts, which highly concentrate the active compounds in green tea.

What is it supposed to do?

Green tea contains a long list of compounds that appear to have all sorts of biological effects, from increasing metabolic rate, to being powerful antioxidants and immune modulators.

The major active compounds in green tea extracts are: polyphenols (catechins) and flavonols. These two major categories are broken down into many subgroups of active compounds such as flavonoids, epigallocatechin gallate, epicatechin gallate, epicatechin, epigallocatechin and tannins, as well as other active constituents, including varying amounts of caffeine.

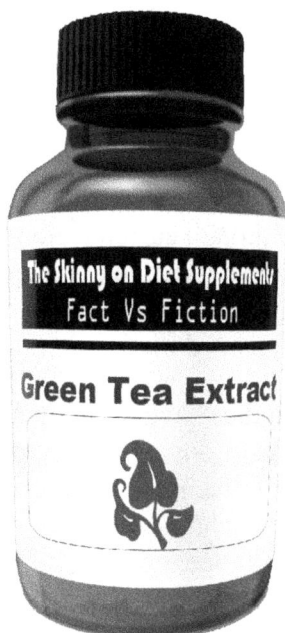

Studies suggest epigallocatechin gallate (EGCG) appears to be the most powerful of the catechins. Some research shows it has up to 100 times greater antioxidant activity than vitamins C and E!

Oxidative stress is associated with a long list of diseases, such as cancer, heart disease, immune suppression, and other pathologies.

From a weight loss point of view, green tea extracts may offer some real benefits to the dieter. Green tea and green tea extracts do contain small amounts of caffeine. Caffeine is known to increase energy levels, help the body to liberate stored body fat for energy, and other functions well known to most people (readers should review the ephedrine/caffeine section for more info on caffeine).

Although caffeine alone has the above properties, recent studies have shown green tea may be superior to simple caffeine for liberating stored body fat as a fuel and may also be superior for energy levels and enhanced metabolic rate.

Studies have found that the catechins in green tea inhibit the enzyme that breaks down norepinephrine (catechol O–methyltransferase), while caffeine inhibits the cyclic AMP degrading enzymes (phosphodiesterases); also green tea extract may have a greater effect on thermogenesis. It should also be highly synergistic when combined with other thermogenic compounds.

Green tea has a wide range of potential health benefits. As mentioned prior, various compounds in green tea extracts act as antioxidants. They may also reduce blood pressure, prevent LDL cholesterol from oxidation, prevent certain forms of cancer, improve immunity, prevent heart disease and control blood sugar.

Epidemiological studies suggest that people who drink green tea have significantly lower risks of many diseases, including cancer, heart disease and stroke. Laboratory studies show that green tea extract protects against, and may be an effective treatment for, many common degenerative diseases as listed above. Green tea catechins are potent antioxidants that provide health benefits beyond their ability to neutralize free radicals.

Heart disease and stroke are associated with a number of risk factors, yet the surprising news is that green tea appears to mitigate many of these risk factors.

Green tea has been shown to lower LDL cholesterol and serum triglyceride levels. The potent antioxidant effects of green tea appear to inhibit the oxidation of LDL cholesterol in the arteries. The oxidation of LDL cholesterol plays a major contributory role in the formation of atherosclerosis.

The formation of abnormal blood clots (thrombosis) is the leading cause of heart attack and stroke, and green tea has been shown to inhibit abnormal blood clot formation as effectively as aspirin. When looking at coagulation risk factors in the blood, green tea specifically inhibits platelet aggregation and adhesion via effects that differ from those of aspirin.

Green tea reduces the risk of arterial blood clotting by two known mechanisms. First, green tea inhibits thromboxane A2 formation, similar to aspirin. Second, green tea inhibits another clotting agent called "platelet activating factor" (PAF).

Reducing thromboxane A2 levels is highly desirable. High thromboxane levels not only cause arterial blood clots, but also cause arterial constriction. The inhibition of thromboxane can prevent a heart attack or a thrombotic stroke.

Green tea also has been shown to elevate levels of HDL, the good cholesterol that helps remove atherosclerotic plaque from arterial walls. Note that aspirin has some anti-thrombotic effects that differ from green tea, such as inhibition of cyclooxygenase. Green tea polyphenols are potent antioxidants, especially in the brain.

Some studies show that the polyphenols most prevalent in green tea (the catechins) are far more potent in suppressing free radicals than vitamins C or E.

Green tea can kill bacteria and appears to promote the growth of friendly bifidobacteria in the intestine while preventing the growth of dangerous intestinal bacteria such as Clostridia and E. coli.

Green tea also appears to be protective to the immune system in cancer patients undergoing radiation or chemotherapy; white blood cell counts appear to be maintained more effectively in cancer patients consuming green tea.

Interestingly, some research suggests green tea lowers leptin levels, a major hormone involved in metabolic rate and other important metabolic effects relating to weight gain or loss. Another potential downside to green tea is that a few animal studies found it also reduced anabolic hormones such as testosterone in rats.

What does the research say?

Because green tea has such a great deal of varied research behind it, this section will stick to research looking directly at weight loss or weight loss related effects.

Several compelling studies involving humans and animals exist for green tea extracts and its potential effects on metabolism.

For example, a Dr. Abdul G. Dulloo, of the University of Geneva in Switzerland, and colleagues (*Am J Clin Nutr*. 1999;70:1040–045 and *Int J Obes Relat Metab Disord*. 2000 Feb;24(2):252–8) measured the 24-hour energy expenditure, respiratory quotient, and urinary excretion of nitrogen and catecholamines in 10 healthy men who received either placebo, caffeine alone, or green tea extract.

Compared with placebo, the green tea group had significantly increased 24-hour energy expenditure, significantly decreased the 24-hour respiratory quotient, and increased 24-hour urinary norepinephrine excretion.

The effects did not appear to be due to the caffeine, since subjects receiving amounts of caffeine similar to that found in green tea (approx 50 mg) had no changes in any of the same measurements. No changes in urinary nitrogen were observed either.

What this translates into is this; the subjects getting the green tea extract had a higher metabolic rate and were using significantly more body fat (beta–oxidation) for fuel which translated into an additional 800 kJ (191

116

kcal) burned over the 24 hour period without any change in urinary nitrogen.

The group getting the caffeine alone did not experience these effects relative to the green tea group, which leads one to believe green tea has its own unique effects beyond that of its caffeine content.

It also suggested that the green tea group burned fat without sacrificing lean body tissue (muscle), which is essential to the dieter for the importance of muscle mass to the metabolism).

In one animal study using mice, green tea was fed to the mice at between 1 and 4% of their diet for 4 months. The study found that the mice receiving the green tea at all levels ate far less food and gained less overall body weight and accumulated less body fat.

On what might be one of the few negative finding of green tea, is a study that found green tea modulated hormone levels in rats. Green tea catechins were given to rats and studied for their acute effects on the rats' endocrine systems.

Interestingly, the researchers found that EGCG, (considered to be the most powerful catechin in green tea), significantly reduced testosterone levels, estradiol, leptin, insulin, insulin–like growth factor–1 (IGF–1), LH, glucose, cholesterol, and triglycerides! They also found that the EGCG, but not other catechins, reduced the growth of the prostate, uterus, and ovary in the rats.

What does the real world say for weight loss?

Most people report a definite added fat loss benefit to adding a green tea extract to their fat loss supplement regimen, but not everyone reports this effect. The reason may be the wide variation in green tea quality seen on the market.

Will Brink's Recommendation

As indicated above, there is a wide range of quality in green tea extracts on the market. Also, manufacturers will often be extracting different compounds and or may concentrate different compounds in the green tea, which may not specifically be what a person wants for weight loss per se.

The truth is that high quality green tea extracts containing high levels of active compounds are expensive and rarely used in the cost-conscious supplement industry. The few human studies done used a green tea extract containing approximately 90 mg of EGCG. People should look for a green tea extract standardized to at least 60% polyphenols with EGCG as a marker compound.

If people want to drink green tea, they will have to down about to 4-10 cups of strong brewed green tea to get those amounts of polyphenols.

As for the study that found green tea lowered hormone levels, I don't put great stock in that as it was injected into the rats at high doses, rats are not people, and no studies to date have found any problems with green tea in humans.

However, athletes and fitness conscious people interested in maximum muscle mass may need to at least keep that possible issue in mind, though I have never had a single person tell me they lost muscle from using green tea extracts.

As for any safety issues, studies have shown people drinking up to 20 cups per day failed to find any significant side effects. Of course, 20 cups of tea is a high dose of caffeine, and typical side effects of high caffeine intakes such as insomnia may occur.

People that combine green tea with other stimulants such as ephedrine and caffeine products need to also adjust for that.

Also, because green tea can "thin" the blood, individuals taking aspirin or other anticoagulant medications should be aware blood clotting times (bleeding time) could be increased, which has both positive or negative ramifications.

GUGGUL LIPIDS

What is it?

Guggul lipids are derived from the guggul plant, also known as Commiphora mukul. Guggul lipids contain active compounds called guggulsterones. Guggul has been used in Indian Ayurvedic medicine for hundreds, perhaps thousands, of years.

What is it supposed to do?

Guggul is best known for its effects on cholesterol and triglyceride levels. It has been used to reduce total cholesterol levels while increasing HDL (the "good" cholesterol) levels. Guggul is also prescribed for weight loss in some Ayurvedic texts.

Regarding for weight loss, guggul is supposed to stimulate the thyroid gland to increase production of thyroid hormones. Thyroid hormone levels are often suppressed in people from certain nutrient deficiencies, long term low calorie intakes, certain diseases, among other factors.

A "slow" thyroid is often a key area of concern for people trying to lose weight. A slow thyroid (often referred to as sub-clinical hypothyroidism) will make it very difficult for a person to lose weight or keep it off long term. There are many health risks associated with an underactive thyroid and guggul may be able to help with that issue.

Companies are selling guggul as a way of possibly increasing thyroid activity and thus making it easier to maintain a higher metabolic rate and improve weight loss.

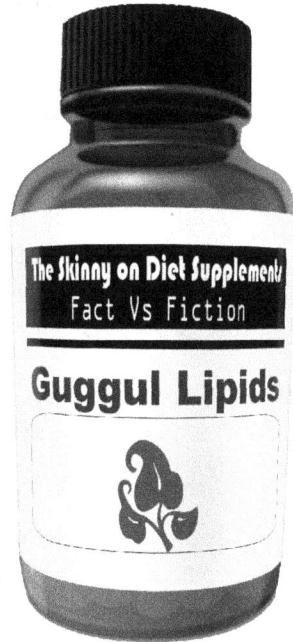

What does the research say?

The majority of research with guggul has focused mainly on its effects on cholesterol levels. Studies on both animals and people suggest guggul is as good, or better, than many of the current lipid reducing drugs currently prescribed to people for reducing cholesterol levels.

The exact mechanism of how guggul achieves its cholesterol lowering effects has not been fully elucidated. It may be related to guggul's supposed effects on the thyroid gland as increased thyroid activity is associated with a reduction in cholesterol levels.

One recent study in mice suggests guggul lowers cholesterol levels by being an antagonist of the FXR receptor, a nuclear hormone receptor that is activated by bile acids. Guggul decreased hepatic cholesterol in mice fed a high-cholesterol diet but was not effective in mice lacking an FXR receptor.

This fact leads researchers to conclude that the inhibition of the FXR receptor is responsible for this herb's cholesterol lowering activity. It's clear however, that guggul has additional effects.

For example, research has shown guggul's lipid lowering activity is related to an increase in LDL breakdown (catabolism). Other possible actions have also been examined. For example, studies with guggul have shown it inhibits certain enzymes involved with cholesterol storage and clearance while increasing the fecal excretion of sterols and bile acids.

Other interesting research suggests guggul may be protective to heart tissue; may have strong anti-inflammatory properties, and for some odd reason, helps cure acne.

As far as weight loss is concerned, little has been done to examine this assertion, although studies from older Indian research mentions weight loss as an effect of the use of guggul lipids. Animal research looking at its effects on the thyroid appears to show thyroid activity increases but human studies are limited or inconclusive.

The one recent study that examined weight loss and guggul combined with other compounds is covered in the next section.

120

What does the real world say for weight loss?

General feedback has been limited and mixed. Most people report no weight loss from taking guggul as the only weight loss nutrient, but very few people have tried it for that use in my experience.

Will Brink's Recommendation

There is no doubt that guggul lipids are an interesting topic with potentially useful applications, such as reducing total cholesterol and triglyceride levels. The lack of modern research examining the effects of guggul on weight loss, combined with lackluster feedback, is a problem but certainly does not mean it is worthless.

The mixed feedback may be due to several of the following issues:

- Thyroid is clearly essential for the regulation of metabolic rate/weight loss, there are many factors that have to be considered, such as GH, UCP's, insulin levels, neurotransmitters, androgens, leptin levels, estrogen levels, and about a hundred other variables, so people are not going to find thyroid output and function as the be all and end all of fat loss. It is definitely one important and worthwhile angle to pursue, however.

- While there is still some debate, guggul does appear to positively affect thyroid output, but the effect may not be great enough to cause weight loss. The thyroid is not the only regulator of the body's metabolism or our ability to lose fat. It's very possible that guggul is useful as part of a formula that combines other nutrients (See next section on guggul and phosphates mixtures for further info).

For people interested in trying this product, research on guggul for reducing cholesterol generally used 50-75 mg of guggulsterones per day in divided doses.

There do not seem to be any major known side effects at this time, however, anything that has the potential to greatly alter thyroid metabolism has the potential for problems in certain people. In particular, if a person has clinical hypothyroidism and is being treated

121

with synthetic thyroid medications, the addition of guggul could have some negative and unknown interactions.

Best advice is for people who are using thyroid meds to avoid guggul products, or be willing to work closely with a doctor to fine tune the dosage of their medications (assuming the guggul has any effects).

For people not using thyroid meds, there should not be any issues. However, I would still recommend cycling this product: 6-8 weeks on and 2-4 weeks off is a good—though unproven—schedule.

What is Slow Thyroid? What you should do if you're already taking thyroid meds?

There has been an ongoing controversy for decades as to whether or not people with sub-clinical hypothyroidism should be treated. Recent studies suggest such people should be treated.

People given thyroid medication with "normal" but low thyroid hormones have shown reductions in cholesterol, improvements in energy and general feelings of well being with no side effects.

One study found that people with hypothyroidism had higher levels of homocysteine which were brought down by thyroid medication (*Ann Intern Med.* 1999 Sep 7;131(5):348–51.). This may also be the case for people with sub-clinical hypothyroidism as well.

If you suspect you have a slow thyroid, you need to find a doctor who treats people with sub-clinical hypothyroidism rather than a doctor who tells you that you don't need it.

If you suspect you have a slow thyroid, your doctor should run a full thyroid panel including: T4, T3, TSH, free T3 and reverse T3. Secondly, make sure you are taking in all the nutrients needed for proper thyroid function, such as kelp (which contains iodine), L–tyrosine (see tyrosine section for more info), zinc, B vitamins, vitamin C, minerals, essential fatty acids, and adequate calories.

Consider using a guggul/phosphate mixture (see next section). Try this strategy for a month or so and get retested.

If that does not work, that is raise your T4 and T3 levels while lowering TSH, you will probably need to have a doctor prescribe a small dose of thyroid medication if they can pinpoint the cause.

What about thyroid medication if you have to go that route?

Again, this has been something of an ongoing controversy in the medical community. There are two main thyroid hormones: thyroxine (T4) and triiodothyronine (T3). T3 possesses about 5 times more activity than T4. The body converts T4 into the more active T3 as needed via an enzyme.

The general logic by most medical professionals in the US has been to give people synthetic T4 (brand name Synthroid) and let the body convert it to T3 as needed. Most docs in the US don't use T3, while it's more commonly prescribed in other countries.

In the old days, doctors prescribed natural desiccated thyroid (brand name Armour Thyroid) which is a mixture of T4 and T3 with other naturally occurring constituents found in thyroid, including the rarely talked about thyroid hormones T1 and T2.

Although many modern traditional doctors have all but dismissed the natural thyroid products, alternative practitioners have found the synthetic thyroid meds did not work as well as the natural Armour thyroid. Many alternative MDs continue to prescribe Armour rather than the synthetic T4 or T3.

Thus a controversy arose as the majority of medical professionals feel simple T4 is fine. Armour thyroid is probably superior, and some studies suggest that a mixture of T4 and T3 is superior to either alone.

For example, a recent study published in the *New England Journal of Medicine* (*NEJM*. 1999; 340: 424–429.) found that a combination of T4 and T3 was more effective than T4 alone for improving mood and neuropsycho logical functions of people with hypothyroidism.

I can also tell you that people who have taken T4 and switched over to Armour often report they feel better and have more energy.

If you need thyroid medication, I suggest the use of the Armour product.

If you already take thyroid meds for some condition, you might want to consider talking to your doctor regarding the use of Armour thyroid.

With sub-clinical hypothyroidism, most docs will start a person off on a half to a whole grain of Armour thyroid. This dose may be higher or lower depending on what the doctor feels is needed however. Each half grain or Armour has approximately 19 mcg of T4 and 4.5 mcg of T3.

Do not undertake the above without proper blood chemistries done or without a medical doctors supervision.

For those on thyroid meds actually diagnosed hypothyroid

Considering how many people are on thyroid medication for hypothyroid conditions, it's amazing how much confusion exists in the medical community on how best to treat people with hypothyroid.

I find many people feel they are often in some sort of battle between themselves and their doctor as to what doses, types, etc of thyroid meds they need.

A book called "*Thyroid Disorders*" written by a Dr Gilbert Daniels, listed as Co- Director of the Thyroid Clinic at Mass General Hospital makes for a good reference guide. The book was published in 2006, so I am assuming he's still there.

The book is written for physicians, specifically for GPs/family physicians vs. specialists. Most of the information would be basic rehash for the people that have already done a lot of research on the topic, and most of what he recommends is in line with the standard recommendations.

However, he makes a few salient points regarding optimizing therapy, which seems to be the major issue for most people.

Unlike many 'traditional' docs out there, Dr Daniels seems fairly open minded. For those looking for a decent reference guide to tests, diagnoses, etc, it's a good little book.

It could also be helpful for when making your case that you are not happy with your current meds/dose, etc and the doc you are working with is resistant. For example, he states:

"Although thyroid function can be precisely, monitored, not all 'optimally treated' patients feel well. For example in one study in which patients were treated with increments of thyroid hormone, those whose T4 dose was increased by 25-50 mcg/d, resulting in a suppressed serum TSH, felt consistently better than those receiving the highest dose at which TSH could be maintained within the normal range. In another community population-based study, patients taking T4 felt psychologically less well than a matched control population."

Possible explanations for the above findings he lists as:

- Some of these patients may have been subtly under treated. When hypothyroid patients remain symptomatic, the T4 dose should be increased until TSH reaches the lower normal range.

(Note, however, he's clear to point out that an intact hyopthalamo-pituitary axis is necessary for TSH to reflect thyroid status appropriately and other measures such as free hormones and symptoms should be used in that situation in addition to TSH)

- The patients may have remained symptomatic because their symptoms were related to other disorders possibly associated with Hashimoto's thyroiditis, such as depression.

- True physiological replacement of thyroid hormone may require both T4 and T3.

- Clinical deterioration after starting T4 therapy should raise the question of concomitant adrenal insufficiency, known as Schmidt's syndrome.

For those people diagnosed as hypothyroid and on thyroid medication, the above info may be of some help if you're still struggling with dose and or type of thyroid medication being used to treat your condition.

Guggul/Phosphate Mixtures

What is it?

I am going to cover guggul/phosphate mixtures as one section as I did with ephedrine/caffeine products. The reason will become apparent shortly. For a full explanation of guggul, see the previous section on guggul lipids. Phosphates are the "P" in ATP. Adenosine triphosphate (ATP) is the often called the "universal energy storage molecule" in the human body.

What is it supposed to do?

Guggul lipids were covered in the previous section, and therefore only a short explanation is needed here. Guggul lipids (containing various guggulsterones) have been shown to reduce cholesterol and triglycerides. They may possibly improve thyroid function, and have other potential health uses.

The role of ATP would take an entire biochemistry text book to cover, so we will narrow our discussion to the topic of weight loss and its possible synergism to guggul and thyroid function.

Even narrowing our discussion of ATP to weight loss and thyroid function is going to get a tad complicated and will need some set up. Bear with me on this as it will be lengthy but worth it.

We all know you have to reduce calories to get the body to lose weight, right? As most people already know from their own diet experience, the body responds to a decrease in calories by slowing down the metabolism. As mentioned in the previous section on guggul lipids, the thyroid gland is a major player in the regulation of metabolic rate.

There are two primary thyroid hormones, which are thyroxine (T4) and triiodothyronine (T3). T3 is about 5 times more active than T4, and this interplay is one of many ways the body regulates metabolism. That is, the body will convert T4 to T3 as needed or block the conversion as needed to speed up or slow down the metabolism in response to caloric intake and other factors.

When the body senses a reduction in calories, there is a reduction in the conversion of the thyroid hormone T4, to the more active T3, thus slowing down the metabolism and potentially reducing the effectiveness of the diet.

This is one of several reasons diets fail to be effective after a short period of time, thus forcing the person to restrict calories even further and beginning a vicious cycle. Therefore, anything that can reduce or delay this reduction in thyroid hormones should have positive effects on fat loss.

Another important point to know about metabolic rate and thyroid hormones; most of the conversion of T4 to T3 takes place in the liver. When a person is well fed they have a high ATP storage.

When we diet, ATP stores decline and the liver appears to be the main sensing organ of this system. If liver ATP declines, the body senses this and adjusts the thyroid output and conversion of T4 to T3 downward, that is to say, the conversion of T4 to T3 is partially dependent on the ATP status of the liver.

Therefore, anything that can maintain liver ATP should fool the system into thinking it is well fed, thus hopefully maintaining adequate thyroid output. This is where the use of phosphates may come in.

Phosphates may allow a person to maintain a higher liver ATP content without eating extra food. Translated, by ingesting phosphates (a non-caloric ATP substrate), it may be possible to maintain liver ATP levels without adding any calories to the diet and the person can maintain a higher metabolism.

Further translated, you take in stuff that can be made into ATP, in order to trick your system into thinking you are eating plenty of food, even though it has no caloric value. Got all that? Go ahead, and read it again, I can wait.

What does the research have to say?

The research on guggul was covered in the previous section on guggul lipids. Several studies using a combination of mixed phosphates (the "P" in ATP) fed to people appeared to show an increase in metabolism and a maintenance of T3 levels in people who were put on a diet.

One study found that when thirty overweight women who participated in 8 week "slimming program" were given supplemental mixed phosphate/mineral tablets, they maintained higher T3 levels and resting metabolic rate over a group not getting the supplement.

However, the actual rate of weight loss was similar in both groups. The study found during the periods of phosphate supplementation, the resting metabolic rate (RMR) increased in addition to the effects on thyroid hormone levels. The study concluded:

"This effect seems to be, at least partly, due to an influence of phosphates on peripheral metabolism of thyroid hormones."

Another study with the long name of "**Effect of Phosphate Supplementation on Metabolic and Neuroendocrine Responses to Exercise and Oral Glucose Load in Obese Women During Weight Reduction**" found essentially the same thing.

The study had thirty six chunky women (BMI 29.5 to 44.0 kg m-2, aged 27 to 45 yrs) participate in the 4 week weight reducing program. They were put on a low calorie diet and given phosphate supplements and were found to have a higher RMR and maintained higher levels of T3 which normally would have dropped with reduced calorie intake.

However, there was little or no difference in weight loss between groups getting the phosphates and those not getting them, and that's an important point. The authors of the study stated:

"In conclusion, the present study confirmed a potential usefulness of phosphate supplementation during energy restriction in obese patients due to its effect on resting metabolic rate. The results did not, however, reveal any major alterations in the metabolic and hormonal responses to exercise or to glucose ingestion in comparison with placebo treatment."

So far, research with phosphates, though interesting and promising, does not seem to show it has effects on weight loss when used as the only supplement. This is the logic behind this discussion of combining guggul and phosphates in one supplement.

A recent study that looked at the combination of guggul and phosphates did in fact seem to find real effects on weight loss.

The study was a prospective, double blind, placebo controlled study involving 18 people. Each person was put on an 1800 calorie diet and workout, done three days per week doing 45 minutes of circuit training and aerobics, which is not very strenuous by most standards.

After six weeks, the study found that the group receiving the guggul/phosphate mixture lost three times more fat than the placebo group or control group (9.4 lbs. of fat lost for the guggul/phosphate group vs 3 lbs. and 2.9 lbs. for placebo and control group respectively) while neither group experienced changes in muscle mass.

These results would suggest that there is a possible synergism between guggul and phosphates, similar in effect to that of ephedrine and caffeine. Of course, EC products work through very different mechanisms than that of the guggul/phosphate product used in this study.

The product used in the study (Metabolic Thyrolean) also contained the ingredients choline, garcinia cambogia, and tyrosine, but the main effect was believed to come from the guggul/phosphate mixture.

The study also found no side effects. An interesting side note is that, the study also looked at something called a Profile of Mood States (POMS), a common psychological test used to test the mood of subjects.

The POMS test found that the people getting the guggul/phosphate formulation were less prone to fatigue and had better mood scores. They just felt better than the other groups not getting the product.

Some research suggests phosphates may improve athletic performance by altering the lactic acid buffering system of the body, but that has been a mixed bag and inconclusive. Unfortunately, the was a small study and the only study that exists for that specific mixture. Additional/larger studies need to be done for truly conclusive answers from a research perspective.

What does the real world say for weight loss?

The feed back for guggul lipids as covered in the previous section has been mixed or disappointing. Feedback for phosphates has been disappointing regarding weight loss, although some people feel they have more energy and strength when using phosphate supplements.

Feedback for the product that combines the two, on the other hand has been generally positive for the most part.

This leads me to believe that neither ingredient alone has enough effect on metabolism to help with weight loss, but together, there may be synergism (The US Patent Office was also convinced enough regarding the idea of a synergistic effect of these two ingredients to award the manufacturer and sponsor of the study, Prolab Nutrition™, a composition patent on the formulation).

Of course, patents are not a guarantee that something works, but if a company goes through the time and expense to protect their findings and product, in may be inferred the information has perceived value.).

Will Brink's Recommendation

Those who wish to read up on the specific guggul/phosphate product used in the study can read the full article on the topic at my web site at BrinkZone.com.

My advice at this time is it's a "might worth a try" supplement. There is decent research behind it, but more is clearly needed specific to this exact mixture. There's been generally good feedback, it's safe, and not terribly expensive.

However, I don't think guggul/phosphate mixtures will prove superior to EC products for fat loss but they (a) may be a particularly good combination with EC based products and (b) may be a good alternative for those who can't tolerate the EC based products.

131

Note: It's my understanding the specific product the study was based on is no longer available. However, there's probably similar formulas and or one can simply make their own by buying the ingredients separately.

HOODIA

What is it?

Hoodia gordonii is a plant in the succulent family that grows in the Kalahari Desert and other parts of Africa. As the story goes, for thousands of years Kalahari Bushmen have been eating this plant to stave off hunger during their long hunting trips.

What is it supposed to do?

As implied above, Hoodia is supposed to have anorectic (appetite suppressing) effects, leading to less food eaten—which means fewer calories ingested. The compound in Hoodia that supposedly has this effect is a steroidal glycoside with the name P57AS3 or simply P57.

Supposedly, the main effect of P57 is to affect nerve cells in the hypothalamus that monitor ATP and perhaps blood glucose.

The result is that the brain is "tricked" into thinking there is enough energy (ATP) in the system and shuts down hunger signals. Direct injections into the brains of rats (poor rats!) using the purified P57 demonstrated that the compound likely has a central (CNS) mechanism of action via the hypothalamus. That's the basic hypothesis anyway.

What does the research say?

Research with Hoodia is limited but moderately compelling. For example, a study entitled "**Increased ATP content/production in the hypothalamus may be a signal for energy-sensing of satiety: studies**

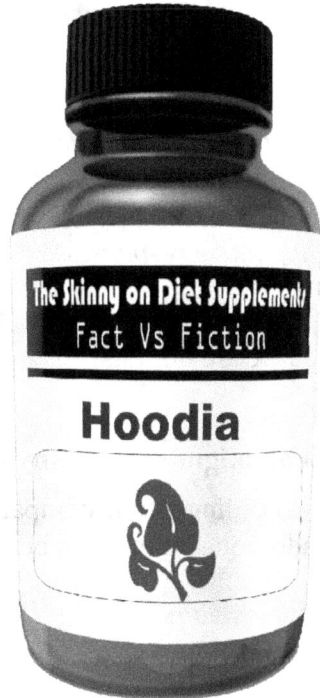

of the anorectic mechanism of a plant steroidal glycoside" (*Brain Res.* 2004 Sep 10;1020(1-2):1–11.) found P57 to be an effective appetite suppressant in rats.

This study found P57 increased the ATP content by up to 150% in hypothalamic neurons of the rats' brains with a reduced 24-h food intake by 40-60%.

The researchers concluded:

"With growing evidence of metabolic or nutrient-sensing by the hypothalamus, ATP may be a common currency of energy sensing, which in turn may trigger the appropriate neural, endocrine and appetitive responses..."

This was done in rats, not humans, and that is an important distinction, as we are not rats!

You might ask: do any human studies exist?

According to one company that claims a patent on Hoodia (see additional comments below) a human study has been done.

They claim:

"In 2001 Phytopharm completed a double-blind, placebo-controlled clinical study in overweight, but otherwise healthy volunteers using an extract of Hoodia gordonii. The large doses of extract caused a statistically significant reduction in the average daily calorie intake. In addition, a statistically significant reduction in body fat content was also observed compared to the placebo group after two weeks."

Problem is, the study does not appear to have been published in any peer reviewed journals, nor is any journal listed on their web site. Taking the manufacturer's word for a study being done and having positive effects (one has to assume at this point it was an 'in-house' study) is essentially worthless for our purposes of examining the research in this section of the book.

A recent published study in humans appears to put a nail in the coffin of hoodia and suggest it may be potentially toxic. This study found not only

134

did 15 days of a hoodia purified extract (HgPE) not reduce food intake in a double blind study in healthy overweight women, it negatively impacted blood pressure (went up), increased heart rate, and elevated some liver function tests.

This study was published in a 2011 addition of the American Journal of Clinical Nutrition ("**Effects of 15-d repeated consumption of Hoodia gordonii purified extract on safety, ad libitum energy intake, and body weight in healthy, overweight women: a randomized controlled trial**") and caused a major company to drop its development of Hoodia as a weight loss supplement.

What does the real world say for weight loss?

Feedback has been limited and hoodia is usually found in mixtures, so difficult to give useful feedback, and it's also well established very little legit Hoodia is found in most products sold anyway (see comments below) so it's near impossible to give feedback on this plant.

Will Brink's Recommendation

There are no published long-term studies on the safety of Hoodia, nor even adequate animal studies to make any conclusive recommendations about it. The short lived study mentioned above suggest Hoodia is neither effective nor safe. The fact that Bushmen have used it for thousands of years in Africa is not exactly legit safety data by any stretch.

My recommendation at this time would be to avoid Hoodia supplements.

Note:

Another issue with Hoodia as it relates to supplements is the issue of quality control; is there even any active p57 in any of the products currently being sold?

A company called Phytopharm supposedly holds the exclusive patents for extracting p57 and some reports suggest there is essentially no p57 in most commercial products.

To add to that, there are no published studies in humans to suggest what a therapeutic dose might be for this compound, although anecdotal reports indicate as much as 1 g, 3 times/day might be needed.

Needless to state, this is a much larger amount than is used in most supplements.

5–HTP

What is it?

5–hydroxytryptophan (5–HTP) is a precursor to the neurotransmitter serotonin. 5–HTP can be produced synthetically, but many supplements contain 5–HTP derived from the Griffonia simplicifolia seed.

What is it supposed to do?

As mentioned above, 5–HTP converts into the neurotransmitter serotonin in both the brain and the peripheral tissues. As most people know, serotonin is a very hot topic and area of research right now due to serotonin's effects on mood, depression, etc.

Serotonin is probably the most studied neurotransmitter since it has been found to be involved in a wide range of psychological and biological functions. Serotonin (also called 5–hydroxytryptamine or 5–HT) is involved with mood, anxiety, and appetite.

Elevated levels of serotonin can cause relaxation and reduced anxiety. Low serotonin levels are associated with low mood, increased anxiety (hence the current popularity of the SSRI drugs such as Prozac and others), and poor appetite control.

This is an extremely abbreviated description of all the functions serotonin performs in the human body—many of which have yet to be fully elucidated—but a full explanation is beyond the scope of this section and unneeded anyway.

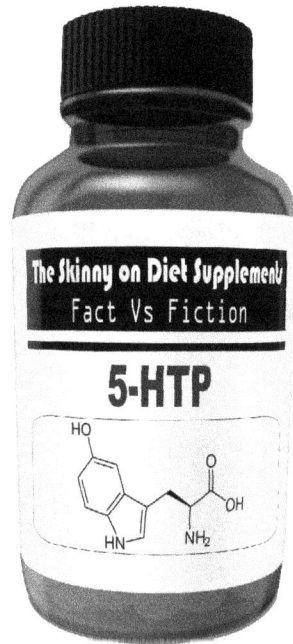

Needless to say, increased brain serotonin levels are associated with an improved ability of people to cope with stress, whereas a decline in serotonin activity is associated with depression and anxiety. Elevated levels of serotonin in the body often result in the relief of depression, as well as substantial reduction in pain sensitivity, anxiety and stress.

It has also been theorized that a diet-induced increase in tryptophan will increase brain serotonin levels, while a diet designed for weight loss (e.g., a diet that reduces calories) may lead to a reduction of brain serotonin levels due to reduced substrate for production and a reduction in carbohydrates.

Many people who reduce their calorie intake in an attempt to lose weight find they are often ill-tempered and more anxious. Reductions in serotonin may be partially to blame here. The basic theory is 5–HTP increases brain serotonin levels which should lead to improved mood states and a reduction in food intakes.

What does the research say?

The research with 5–HTP for weight loss specifically is interesting and compelling, but spotty. The research looking at mood elevation is more extensive.

Since this book concerns itself with weight loss only, I will focus on the studies that examined weight loss with 5–HTP. One study done with overweight Type–2 diabetics (*Int J Obes Relat Metab Disord.* 1998 Jul;22(7):648–54.) found patients receiving 750 mg per day of 5–HTP:

"significantly decreased their daily energy intake, by reducing carbohydrate and fat intake, and reduced their body weight"

compared to the placebo group.

Another study done by the same group of researchers out of Italy (*Am J Clin Nutr.* 1992 Nov;56(5):863–7) called "**Eating behavior and adherence to dietary prescriptions in obese adult subjects treated with 5-hydroxytryptophan**" found similar results.

In this study 20 obese patients were randomly assigned to receive either 900 mg per day of 5–HTP or a placebo. The study was a double-blind design that ran for two consecutive six week periods.

For the first six weeks, no specific diet was prescribed. For the second six week period, a specific reduced-calorie diet was recommended.

According to this study:

"Significant weight loss was observed in 5–HTP-treated patients during both periods. A reduction in carbohydrate intake and a consistent presence of early satiety were also found. These findings together with the good tolerance observed suggest that 5–HTP may be safely used to treat obesity."

Finally, an earlier study done by the same group (*J Neural Transm.* 1989;76(2):109–17) found more or less the same results with obese women and concluded:

"The administration of 5-hydroxytryptophan resulted in no changes in mood state but promoted typical anorexia-related symptoms, decreased food intake and weight loss during the period of observation."

The major side effect reported in some of the studies with 5–HTP is nausea which appears to go away with time. The total weight loss in these studies, although statistically significant (vs. placebo) are not huge, generally in the 10 lbs. range, give or take, which is due to appetite reduction vs. an increase in metabolic rate.

What does the real world say for weight loss?

Real world feedback has generally been lackluster. The issue may simply be one of dose (see below), or other factors.

Will Brink's Recommendation

Although 5–HTP generally looks good as a potential supplement for weight loss, there are many points and caveats that have to be made that may tip the balance toward <u>not</u> recommending it. So far, there does not appear to be any toxicity concerns with 5–HTP but I am still wary.

One issue is the peripheral conversion of 5–HTP which does not reach the brain. It works like this: some of the 5–HTP converts to serotonin before it reaches the brain. The brain does not let the serotonin through a permeable membrane called the "blood brain barrier" which acts as a sort of selective filter for the brain.

The theory being then that the body has to deal with excess levels of serotonin which could lead to side effects.

However, to date, no major side effects have been reported. A review on the potential toxicity of 5–HTP (*Toxicol Lett*. 2004 Apr 15;150(1):111–22) stated:

"...no definitive cases of toxicity have emerged despite the worldwide usage of 5–HTP for last 20 years, with the possible exception of one unresolved case of a Canadian woman."

As some may already know, the amino acid L–tryptophan was removed from the market in 1989 due to an outbreak of eosinophilia–myalgia syndrome (EMS) that was traced to a contaminated synthetic L–tryptophan from a single manufacturer.

According to the aforementioned review above however:

"Extensive analyses of several sources of 5–HTP have shown no toxic contaminants similar to those associated with L–Tryptophan, nor the presence of any other significant impurities."

The bottom line here is that 5–HTP appears safe, but there are theoretical reasons it may not be long-term. People already taking SSRI drugs should probably not combine 5–HTP with those drugs as the interaction between the two has not been well explored.

Some of my other concerns are that all the studies above came from the same group of researchers. It's essential that another lab confirms their findings, as it has often been the case that other researchers are unable to replicate the effects a lab has produced.

Finally, as I have said over and over in this book, read the labels, people! Most of the 5–HTP products are far too under dosed to have any effects. If the product does not contain what the studies found effective, don't purchase it!

As always, dosage is the critical issue here: those last 3 studies used 750 mg/d, 900 mg/d, and 8 mg/kg/d (so 800 mg/d for a 100 kg person).

Most OTC supplement doses range in the 5-100 mg range either as part of a blend, or taken straight. For people that want to try, start with 200 mg three times per day before meals and work up to 300 mg X 3 per day. At these higher doses, nausea for the first 6 weeks has been reported in the literature.

This doesn't seem to be an issue however, unless you take over 200 mg/day. 5–HTP gets a "might be worth a try" rating with some caveats already mentioned.

Possible drug interactions to be aware of

If you are treated with SSRI's, MAOI's and some types of pain medications, you should not take 5-HTP without first talking to your healthcare provider.

Antidepressants medications that can interact with 5-HTP include:

SSRIs: Citalopram (Celexa), escitalopram (Lexapro), fluvoxamine (Luvox), paroxetine (Paxil), fluoxetine (Prozac), sertraline (Zoloft)

Tricyclics: Amitriptyline (Elavil), nortryptyline (Pamelor), imipramine (Tofranil)

Monoamine oxidase inhibitors (MAOIs):

Phenelzine, (Nardil), tranylcypromine (Parnate)

Nefazodone (Serzone)

Certain types of pain medications:

Tramadol (Ultram) -- Tramadol, used for pain control may also increase serotonin levels too much if taken in combination with 5-HTP.

Triptans (used to treat migraines): 5-HTP can increase the risk of side effects, including serotonin syndrome, when taken with these medications:

Naratriptan (Amerge)

Rizatriptan (Maxalt)

Sumatriptan (Imitrex)

Zolmitriptan (Zomig)

Source: Medline
http://www.nlm.nih.gov/medlineplus/druginfo/natural/794.html

HYDROXYCITRIC ACID (HCA)

What is it?

Hydroxycitric acid (HCA) is derived from the fruit of the Garcinia cambogia plant, a plant found in South Asia.

What is it supposed to do?

It's claimed that HCA is able to block the conversion of excess carbohydrate calories into stored body fat. HCA blocks an enzyme called ATP–citrate lyase. This enzyme is involved in the early stages of fat synthesis.

By blocking this enzyme, in theory, more carbohydrate calories will be stored as glycogen in muscle and liver tissue while fewer excess calories from carbohydrates will be stored as body fat.

The basic metabolic rule is, when the body tops off its stores of glycogen (stored muscle sugars) any excess carbohydrates will be burned off as heat (i.e. thermic effects) and stored as body fat. ATP–citrate lyase is a key enzyme in that system. HCA is marketed to a lesser degree as an appetite suppressant. It may also enhance thermogenesis, which is the production of heat from food and may be beneficial in reducing total cholesterol and LDL ("bad" cholesterol) levels.

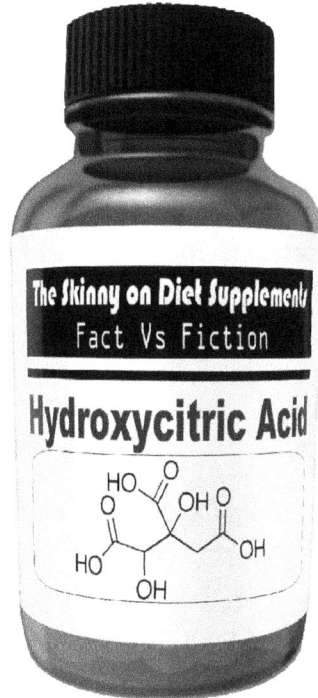

What does the research say?

In-vitro (test tube) research has shown that HCA blocks ATP–citrate lyase. In animals, HCA appears to be a legitimate weight loss agent. Several decades of animal research has shown HCA to be a good appetite suppressant, presumably by sending the fullness (satiety) signal to the brain after changes in glycogen status in the liver.

Rats and mice given HCA eat less food and gain less body fat from the food they ingest. As we all know, the metabolism of rats and humans are quite different so the positive animal studies may not be duplicated or possible in humans.

What does the real world say for weight loss?

HCA is a product that has been around for quite a while. The vast majority of feedback regarding weight loss with people using HCA has been negative in my experience. At higher doses, some people do feel HCA has a mild anorectic (appetite suppressing) effect.

Will Brink's Recommendation

The use of HCA for weight/fat loss may seem bleak from the above discussion, but I actually hold out some hope for this product. HCA may have had poor feedback and results because of several factors. One factor may be simple dose. Most weight loss formulas containing HCA don't have enough for a measurable response. HCA probably needs to be taken in the multi gram range (1000 to 5000 mg) in divided doses per day to have any effects, if it is to have any effects at all.

I would consider 1000 mg per day of the more absorbable forms to be a minimum daily intake. Up until recently, HCA products were in calcium-HCA form and this form may not be very absorbable. Newer HCA types can be found as potassium and potassium/magnesium forms of HCA salts. Unfortunately, the dose needed to have an effect (if there is any effect) is expensive.

HCA appears to be a very safe supplement with no known side effects. People who wish to try HCA should start with 250 mg of HCA 30-40 minutes prior to a meal three times a day and increase the dose until an effect is observed.

144

INSULIN POTENTIATORS

What are they?

There are a variety of different agents that are used in weight loss supplements for controlling blood sugar and enhancing insulin sensitivity. The most common ones are: Gymnema sylvestre extract, fenugreek extract, cinnamon extract, d–pinitol, and alpha–lipoic acid.

What are they supposed to do?

Obesity is linked to the development of metabolic syndrome (a.k.a Syndrome X) and insulin resistance (*N Engl J Med.* 2004 Jun 3;350(23):2362–74.) which predispose to type 2 diabetes. Agents that enhance glycemic control have an obvious role in improving glucose metabolism and other parameters associated with hyperglycemia/insulin resistance: elevated blood pressure, serum lipids, and markers of inflammation (C-reactive protein).

What does the research say?

- *Gymnema sylvestre*
  Gymnema sylvestre is an herb used in Ayurvedic medicine: when chewed, the leaves reduce the ability to detect sweetness. The leaves contain a variety of compounds known as saponins: one of these, dubbed "gymnemic acid" has been demonstrated to decrease blood glucose levels in human and animal studies, and to enhance the secretion of insulin in in-vitro (tissue and cell culture) models (*Diabetes Care.* 2003 Apr;26(4):1277–94).

  A study in rats also suggested it can inhibit maltose absorption in the small intestine (*World J Gastroenterol.* 2001 Apr;7(2):270–4.).

- *Fenugreek extract*
  Fenugreek leaves and seeds have been used medicinally since ancient times. Current research suggests that fenugreek extracts have both hypoglycemic and anti-hyperlipidemic properties. These activities have been linked to the presence of an unusual amino acid: 4–hydroxyisoleucine (4–OH–Ile). In animal models, 4–OH–Ile administration resulted in significant improvements in blood lipid profiles (*Bioorg Med Chem Lett*. 2006 Jan 15;16(2):293–6.), improves glucose-stimulated insulin secretion/reduces hyperglycemia (*Am J Physiol*. 1999 Oct;277(4 Pt 1):E617–23.), and enhances insulin sensitivity (*Am J Physiol Endocrinol Metab*. 2004 Sep;287).

  There have been several small, uncontrolled studies in humans with Type 2 and Type 1 diabetes that suggest improved glycemic control and reductions in serum triglycerides and LDL ("bad" cholesterol) with fenugreek seed powder, but further research is needed to confirm these effects. 4–OH–Ile has also been shown to enhance post-exercise glycogen synthesis in a study on trained male cyclists at a dose of 2 mg/kg (*Amino Acids*. 2005 Feb;28(1):71–6.).

- *D–pinitol*
  D–pinitol is 3–O–methyl–D–chiro–inositol; a type of sugar molecule that occurs in a variety of legumes. In animal experiments, it improves glucose uptake by mimicking the effects of insulin, rather than enhancing insulin secretion (*Br J Pharmacol*. 2000 Aug;130(8):1944–8.). At a dose of 1.0g/day (0.5g, 2x/day), d–pinitol was shown to enhance creatine uptake and retention during a 3 day loading protocol in human volunteers, similar to combinations of creatine with carbohydrate and carbohydrate/protein (*JEP*. 2001;4(4);41–47.).

- *Cinnamon extract*
  Cinnamon—either as ground bark of Cinnamomum cassia or an aqueous extract—is the subject of intensive research as a natural agent for blood glucose control. Cinnamon and/or cinnamon extracts have been shown to reduce glucose levels in animal models of diabetes (*Phytother Res*. 2005 Mar;19(3):203–6.).

146

In addition, cinnamon prevented the development of insulin resistance in rats fed a high fructose diet (*Horm Metab Res*. 2004 Feb;36(2):119–25.). One of the active compounds, methylhydroxy chalcone polymer (MHCP), acts as an insulin mimic, and increased glucose metabolism over 20 times in an in-vitro assay using cultured adipocytes (fat cells) (*J Am Coll Nutr*. 2001 Aug;20(4):327–36.).

The efficacy of cinnamon supplements for improving serum glucose and lipids for people with Type–2 diabetes was demonstrated by a recent study (*Diabetes Care*. 2003 Dec;26(12):3215–8.). The researchers gave either placebo capsules or supplements containing 1, 3, or 6 grams of ground cinnamon to 60 people with Type–2 diabetes for 40 days.

Substantial reductions in fasting serum glucose (18-29%), triglycerides (23-30%), LDL ("bad") cholesterol (7-27%), and total cholesterol (12-26%) were seen at all three levels of cinnamon intake.

- *Alpha–lipoic acid*
  Alpha–lipoic acid is another nutrient that may improve insulin sensitivity and glucose disposal. Although known as a powerful antioxidant, alpha–lipoic acid's abilities as a potential "insulin mimicking" compound have only recently been discovered.

This compound has been used extensively in Germany and other countries to treat certain complications associated with diabetes.

To date, the majority of research with alpha–lipoic acid has been done on true diabetics.

Regardless, alpha–lipoic acid has been shown to stimulate insulin activity and to reduce insulin resistance in many clinical trials with diabetes sufferers. In fact, in one study of adult diabetic patients, alpha–lipoic acid increased the cellular uptake and oxidation (burning) of glucose by about 50%.

The optimal dosage of alpha–lipoic acid for increasing glucose uptake into muscle appears to be approximately 600 mg per day spread out over two to three meals.

Whether or not alpha–lipoic acid turns out to be the greatest thing since sliced bread for athletes, it is certainly a nutrient that diabetics and the 70-80 million insulin resistant Americans should consider using on a regular basis along with the other nutrients previously mentioned in this section. In healthy humans, it can even improve uptake of creatine monohydrate in skeletal muscle (*Int J Sport Nutr Exerc Metab*. 2003 Sep;13(3):294–302.)

What does the real world say for weight loss?

In OTC diet supplements, these agents are used in combination with other nutrients, so the individual effects are difficult to evaluate. Furthermore, they are frequently under dosed, which limits their therapeutic utility.

Will Brink's Recommendation

So what do all of these nutrients have in common? They all lack any solid research looking directly at weight loss! 2 + 2 rarely = 4 in the human body. Be that as it may, while no one ever lost weight with the simple addition of these nutrients to their diets, they may be useful to a fat loss program by enhancing the effects of diet and exercise on insulin sensitivity and glycemic control.

If the use of these supplements helps with weight loss via its effects on glycemic control, I would expect the effects to be mild at best. Anyone who sees an ad with any of these nutrients being pushed for weight loss and promising "pounds will just melt off!" is lying to you.

What else is new in the weight loss supplement industry?!

LIPOTROPICS

What are they?

There are many nutrients that can be considered "lipotropic." Probably the best known nutrients people associate with the term are inositol and choline. However, nutrients such as methionine, betaine, niacin, lipase, and various herbs such as milk thistle, are also referred to as lipotropic nutrients.

Some of the lipotropic products are naturally occurring in the human body (e.g. lipase) while some are amino acids (e.g. methionine) and others may be derived from herbs (e.g. milk thistle) or vitamins such as niacin.

What is it supposed to do?

"Lipotropic" is a catch-all term to include any nutrient(s) that can help the body both prevent the storage of fat while assisting the body to detoxify wastes and excrete toxins. Lipotropics generally work within the liver and digestive system. Lipotropics may help to emulsify fat, some may help to increase bile release, while still others may prevent fat absorption, to name a few possible mechanisms of the lipotropic nutrients.

It is a large group of nutrients with diverse and different mechanisms of action with a similar goal.

What does the research say?

As you can plainly see, the number of nutrients considered lipotropic makes it difficult to look at specific studies. Many of the lipotropic nutrients have been found to have potential medicinal uses, such as niacin being recommended for lowering cholesterol, but the lipotropic concept for weight loss is pretty much uncharted territory as far as real research is concerned.

What does the real world say for weight loss?

Do you have to ask :-) ?

Will Brink's Recommendation

Lipotropics, such as inositol and choline, have been around forever as weight loss supplements and they don't do a bloody thing for weight loss.

Some may, in fact, be helpful ingredients in a weight loss formula for various reasons, but used alone are not effective weight loss products.

However, it's a broad category of products. For example, choline is a precursor to certain neurotransmitters and may have an additive effect to some formulas, but it's a tough thing to prove. Betaine may help improve digestion, and that can be beneficial to certain individuals who are deficient in stomach acids and have associated digestive problems often improved by the use of betaine and digestive enzymes.

Many studies have shown the cholesterol lowering abilities of niacin, but whether it affects weight loss is debatable and unproven by medical science.

My general recommendation at this time: If a lipotropic nutrient is found in some weight loss formula that has other effective ingredients, no harm is done. It may or may not help—my guess is probably not. Products sold exclusively as lipotropic formulas (i.e. inositol and choline supplements) are unlikely to have any appreciable effects on weight loss. It's also impossible to give a run down of the possible side effects of the lipotropic nutrients as there are so many of them, often working through totally different mechanisms.

For example, the side effects of too much betaine could cause a stomach ache and heart burn. The side effects of high dose niacin are totally different and range from flushing to burning skin sensations. As a rule however, none of the general lipotropic nutrients currently sold as such would be considered toxic.

L–Tyrosine

What is it?

Tyrosine is an amino acid which is an essential precursor or "building block" to the neurotransmitters responsible for maintaining metabolic rate. L–tyrosine is the direct precursor to stimulatory neurotransmitters such as epinephrine and norepinephrine (i.e. adrenaline and noradrenaline) as well as certain thyroid hormones and dopamine. In other words, L–tyrosine is a precursor to important stimulants to the metabolism. It is also considered a non-carbohydrate ATP substrate.

Tyrosine is a precursor to CCK (see section on glycomacropeptide for a discussion on the effects of CCK). High amounts of tyrosine are found in foods high in protein. The body can make tyrosine from the amino acid phenylalanine.

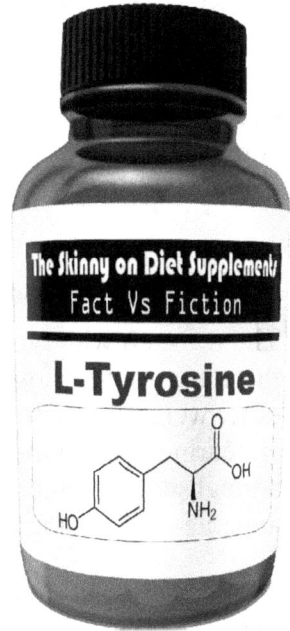

What is it supposed to do?

As the above would imply, tyrosine is an important amino acid for maintaining a higher metabolic rate. As people reduce their calories during a diet, less tyrosine is available to make the natural stimulants to metabolism. Therefore, the metabolism slows down making it harder to lose weight.

Fewer building blocks for stimulants results in a slower metabolism. This is an overly simple explanation, but you get the idea.

This may be one more way the body has built its own safety net to respond to fewer calories being eaten. By taking L–tyrosine as a supplement you supply the building blocks to these important neurotransmitters responsible for maintaining metabolic rate.

This may allow the dieter to bypass some of the metabolic down-regulation from a reduced calorie diet, thus maintaining a higher metabolic rate making weight loss easier and avoiding plateaus.

Tyrosine may also act as an anorectic (appetite suppressing) supplement via its effects on CCK and other mechanisms. Tyrosine is also sold as a mild stimulant and some feel it may be useful for depression. Under stressful conditions, food sources and phenylalanine-to-tyrosine conversion may be inadequate to maintain the essential neurotransmitters needed for optimal performance.

What does the research have to say?

The research with tyrosine as a weight loss agent is limited. However, there are studies showing tyrosine can potentiate the anorectic effects of other weight loss compounds, such as phenylpropanolamine and ephedrine making their effects more prolonged and effective. Several animal studies demonstrated that tyrosine is a powerful potentiator of the appetite-suppressing qualities of the ephedrine-based supplements.

Although human studies using tyrosine mixed with ephedrine are limited, one would expect similar results as found in animals. Because of the extreme complexity of human metabolism and appetite control, effects in people may not be as dramatic as those seen with animals.

Tyrosine does not appear to increase the thermogenic effects of the ephedrine/caffeine products, but works at the level of the brain to reduce food intake and maintain the availability of stimulatory neurotransmitters. There is research suggesting that the positive effects of ephedrine and other compounds are actually limited by the availability of L–tyrosine.

One area tyrosine shines in the research relates to its effects on mental acuity and stress. The military has been particularly interested in tyrosine for use with troops. Tyrosine may also have direct applications to athletes in rigorous training susceptible to Over Training Syndrome (OTS).

152

Several studies done by the US Army found animals given supplemental L–tyrosine were more resistant to cold temperatures than those not getting the amino acid. Studies with humans given supplemental L–tyrosine have found improved cognitive function when subjected to cold temperatures. One recent study found that 21 cadets fed 2 grams of tyrosine a day, then subjected to a demanding military combat training course, showed reduced effects of stress and fatigue on cognitive task performance.

Several studies have found tyrosine to be a stress fighting nutrient that may counter some of the negative effects of prolonged sleeplessness. As a further test of tyrosine's efficacy, 36 Navy SEALs ingested L–tyrosine during Winter Warfare training. Either tyrosine or a placebo was consumed by the men, who were then exposed to temperatures as low as -10° F.

The study found L–tyrosine prevented the decline in mental acuity common to extreme cold conditions in the SEALs who received the supplement.

At least one study found L–tyrosine reduced levels of the catabolic (muscle wasting) hormone cortisol, and this effect is a major plus to both soldiers and athletes alike.

Studies done by the Naval Aerospace Medical Research Laboratory, Massachusetts Institute of Technology (MIT), and The US Army suggest L–tyrosine may be useful in counteracting stress-related performance decrement and mood deterioration:

- By preventing various forms of stress induced brain depletion of cat echolamines (adrenaline), especially norepinephrine.

- By helping to sustain brain norepinephrine levels which are closely related to stress-induced performance decrements.

- By increasing depleted brain norepinephrine levels and minimizing (or reversing) stress-induced performance decrement.

Showing just how complex human metabolism is, one study found tyrosine increased appetite in women with anorexia. What this shows however is that tyrosine's general anti-stress effects are probably causing the effect.

Several recent studies suggest tyrosine may improve exercise tolerance, treat mild depression, and a host of other positive effects, but this comes as no surprise considering tyrosine's role in metabolism as explained above.

What does the real world say for weight loss?

Because few if any people take tyrosine for weight loss alone, feedback is limited. However, many people feel the addition of tyrosine to various weight loss "stacks" is helpful. Many athletes also feel taking tyrosine prior to exercise has a mild stimulating effect. People often report a general improvement in mood when taking L–tyrosine.

Will Brink's Recommendation

Tyrosine is probably a classic example of a supplement that alone has little effect on weight loss, but when combined with other nutrients, may have synergistic properties.

The evidence that tyrosine potentiates the effects of the EC-based products is certainly compelling enough to warrant using it.

Some weight loss formulas already contain tyrosine but often not enough to have the desired results. In general, a minimum dose is 1000 mg per day although higher amounts are not uncommon. Studies that have found positive effects with tyrosine have used considerably more, ranging from 2000 mg (2 g) to 15000 mg (15 g) daily.

Tyrosine is not a particularly expensive supplement so adding tyrosine to other weight loss formulas is not difficult. Tyrosine is not known to have any serious side effects.

However, because it's a mild stimulant and works at the level of the central nervous system, people using MAO inhibitors, pregnant women, people with high blood pressure, and people sensitive to stimulants, should avoid high doses of tyrosine.

154

People who wish to try tyrosine should try 500-1000 mg two to three times a day on an empty stomach 30-40 minutes prior to meals for best results.

It can also be taken prior to a workout for added energy. The combination of a cup of strong black coffee and a few grams of tyrosine is a great pre-workout mixture used by many athletes "in the know."

Foods high in Tyrosine

- Meat sources including fish, chicken, and pork

- Whole grains, wheat, and oats

- Dairy products such as milk, cheese and yogurt

- Fruits such as avocados and bananas

- Legumes, beans and nuts such as almond, lima beans, sesame seeds and pumpkin seeds

Possible drug interactions to be aware of

If you are currently being treated with any of the following medications, you should not use tyrosine supplements without first talking to your health care provider.

Monoamine Oxidase Inhibitors (MAOIs) -- Tyrosine may cause a severe increase in blood pressure in people taking the antidepressant medications known as MAOIs. This rapid increase in blood pressure (also called "hypertensive crisis") can lead to a heart attack or stroke. For this reason, people taking MAOIs should avoid foods and supplements containing tyrosine. MAOIs include:

Isocarboxazid (Marplan)

Phenelzine (Nardil)

Tranylcypromine (Parnate)

Selegiline

Thyroid hormone -- Tyrosine is a precursor to thyroid hormone, so it might raise levels too high when taken with synthetic thyroid hormones.

Levodopa(L-dopa) -- No one should take tyrosine at the same time as levodopa, a medication used to treat Parkinson's disease because levodopa may interfere with the absorption of tyrosine.

Drug Interactions:

LevodopaMAO InhibitorsMorphine

Source:
http://www.umm.edu/altmed/articles/tyrosine-000984.htm

156

MEDIUM CHAIN TRIGLYCERIDES

What are they?

Medium Chain Triglycerides (MCTs) are a type of lipid (fat). The length and structure of MCTs are different than the long chain fatty acids that are found in the normal diet. MCTs are technically saturated fats that are 8-10 carbons long, as opposed to long chain fatty acids which have 16, 18, or more carbons.

MCTs are derived from the fractioning of other oils, usually coconut oil.

What are they supposed to do?

MCTs are fats with some unique biological properties from that of other lipids. They were originally designed for use with people with digestive disorders that caused malabsorption of long chain fatty acids.

MCTs are absorbed and utilized more efficiently than other fats. The long chain fatty acids we all know and love to eat must be transported in small fat-containing globs known as chylomicrons and then passed through the lymph system. MCTs, on the other hand, are transported through the small intestine into the portal blood and go directly to the liver to be burned as energy, thus bypassing the normal route for fats.

MCTs can also bypass the carnitine shuttle system (see section on carnitine for more info) and can enter the mitochondria directly to be oxidized, or "burned," as energy.

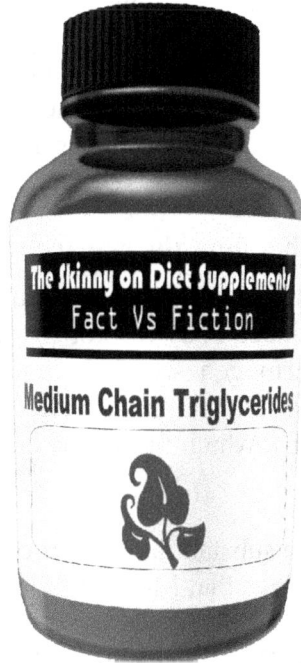

This is one of several reasons MCTs are less likely to be stored as body fat than long chain fatty acids.

MCTs may also increase thermogenesis (heat production) and preserve muscle mass during certain catabolic (muscle wasting) states such as cancer, burns, post surgical, HIV, and other ailments where trauma or disease contributes to a loss of muscle mass.

MCT oil is often marketed to athletes as a sports nutrition supplement as it is a calorie dense energy source less likely to end up as body fat. MCTs are also sold as a weight loss supplement by some companies.

What does the research say?

MCTs have demonstrated a wide variety of effects in animals leading to reduced body fat storage and additional energy being lost as heat (i.e. thermogenesis). In both human and animal research, MCTs seem to increase the thermic effect of food and increase daily energy expenditure (EE); which means the energy is lost as heat rather than stored as body fat.

The substantial number of studies with animals would lead one to believe that MCTs may be a great dieting and fat loss aid for people.

There are also studies showing that in severe catabolic states, such as burns, and certain types of cancer, MCTs are helpful for maintaining nitrogen balance and muscle mass. A handful of human studies have shown the energy expenditure after eating MCTs is higher than for other types of fat, which would suggest that over time the use of MCTs should help with weight loss.

Nonetheless, the studies that have looked directly at the use of MCTs for weight loss are generally disappointing (e.g., there's an effect but it's minimal or there's no effect) or contradictory in humans. In general, most studies seem to find a trend toward weight loss with MCTs, but the effect isn't very impressive.

Why?

Some research suggests MCTs have a more pronounced effect on the release of the fat storing hormone insulin than other fats as well as having other effects that might counter its positive influence on fat loss. MCTs may have some sort of biphasic dual effects that cancel each other out.

One review paper on the topic theorized the reasons for this lack of effect:

"Findings in support of the opinion (lower energy density, control of satiety, rapid intrahepatic delivery and oxidation rates, poor adipose tissue incorporation) may be invalidated by counteracting data (stimulation of insulin secretion and of anabolic-related processes, increased de novo fatty acid synthesis, induced hypertriglyceridemia).

The balance between these two opposing influences depends on the composition (energy intake, nature of ingredients, MCT/LCT ratio, octanoate/decanoate ratio) and duration of the regimen."

Translated, the positive effects of MCTs (increased burning of fats, decreases in hunger, the reduced likelihood of MCTs being made into body fat, etc.) may be offset by some potential negatives. Those negatives may be an increased release of the fat storage hormone insulin, an increase in the production of triglycerides, and other factors.

The net effect may be no fat is lost, at least in humans, though more research is needed for definitive answers.

MCTs does have genuine medical uses where digestion of fats and various liver problems exist, as well as having possible anti-catabolic (muscle sparing) effects in hospitalized patients.

What does the real world say for weight loss?

MCTs are a supplement that just never took off with people. Athletes have used the products to one extent or another for many years, but MCTs have never been very popular in the sports nutrition arena either.

The general feedback is neither very exciting nor very compelling for athletes or people trying lose weight.

Will Brink's Recommendation

MCTs are a classic example of what looks good on paper not always panning out in the real world. It's not that MCTs are of no potential use to the dieter, but in healthy people, they just don't seem to have dramatic effects.

There are drawbacks to using MCTs: in many people, they cause stomach upset. Also, they can cause an odd, scratchy sensation in the back of the throat. As they contain no essential fatty acids (EFAs) a person still needs to take in additional fat to avoid any EFA deficiencies. Nor do MCTs contain fat soluble vitamins such Vitamin E, D, and K essential to human health.

Some studies find they may impact blood lipids negatively, other studies don't find that effect.

In theory, MCTs should be helpful to a weight loss diet but, in practice, they are neither needed nor all that effective in healthy people.

There are no serious side effects of using MCTs, but as they are not a normal part of the human diet in any appreciable amounts, long term effects in healthy people is questionable in my view.

People interested in using MCTs should add a few teaspoons a day to their diet and work their way up to several tablespoons per day over a few weeks. MCT's are a "might be worth a try" type product, but my personal view at this time – based on both the studies and experiences since they were introduced as a dietary supplement two decades or so – is there's better places in your diet to use fat calories and spend your hard earned money.

What about coconut oil?

Coconut oil has become a popular weight loss supplement, with promises of everything from a cancer cure to making one better looking. OK, I'm exaggerating, but the claims for coconut oil are extensive and generally overstated to sell coconut oil…specific to weight loss, the fat from coconut oil is prominently from MCTs (hence why this side bar is following the MCT section) and comments on coconut oils–as it pertains specifically to weight loss–would be the same as for MCTs.

Coconut oil is not pure MCTs however. The impressive write-ups people see on coconut oil and weight loss, will use cited studies from MCT research, not coconut oil specifically, which is both scientifically unsound and intellectually dishonest.*

There's actually very little research done with coconut oil specifically for weight loss in humans, and again, effects are either not very impressive or is contradictory.

Bottom line on coconut oil is, as saturated fats go, it's a healthy choice, may have some health benefits, and if the effects of studies from MCTs do apply to coconut oil, mild effects on weight loss at best.

However, it's no miracle fat nor miracle diet aid, and people have to still keep track of where it fits in an overall nutrition plan in terms of total calories added, fat calories added, and how much one wants to replace other potential beneficial fats (e.g., fish oils, olive oil, etc.) with coconut oil.

* But what else is new in the diet/diet supplement industry??!

Note of interest about MCTs:

One product that might have real promise, however, is something called a structured lipid, which is a hybrid combination of MCTs and omega–3 fatty acids joined together. In the research, this looks like a great supplement with some interesting properties. To my knowledge, structured lipids have never been marketed as a commercial product for use by athletes or dieters.

OCTOPAMINE

What is it?

Octopamine is chemically related to synephrine, and is found in Citrus aurantium extracts (see synephrine section for more info on Citrus aurantium). In insects, it functions as a neurotransmitter similar to norepinephrine (noradrenaline) in mammals, but it's unclear if it plays a role in human or other mammals.

The Skinny on Diet Supplements
Fact Vs Fiction

Octopamine

What is it supposed to do?

Like synephrine, octopamine is a beta–3 agonist (*Comp Biochem Physiol C Toxicol Pharmacol.* 2000.). Binding to the receptor increases lipolyis (i.e., breakdown of fats) and thermogenesis by stimulating the production of cyclic AMP by adenylate cyclase (see Forskolin section for additional info on cyclic AMP).

What does the research say?

There isn't any research on humans that demonstrates weight or fat loss that we can go on; and very little research on animals. A single study, **"Moderate weight lowering effect of octopamine treatment in obese Zucker rats"** demonstrated a 19% reduction in body weight gain (not weight loss) after being given injections of octopamine (*J Physiol Biochem.* 2003 Sep;59(3):175-82.).

A word about the way the octopamine was given to the rats: needless to state, a compound that's injected may not have the same effects as one that's taken orally—and vice versa. Limited digestion, absorption or

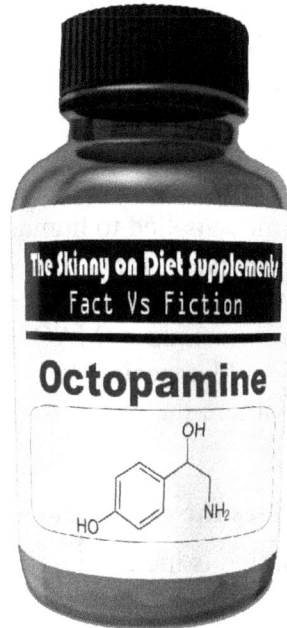

degradation by the liver can limit how much of an oral dose actually reaches the bloodstream and target cells/tissues. So you can't assume that the effects you get when you swallow a compound will be identical to the effects seen when you inject it. No surprise there...

This could be the case with octopamine. According to a small study in humans conducted in 1975, a considerable amount of octopamine taken orally is broken down during "first pass" metabolism by enzymes in the gut (*Eur J Clin Pharmacol.* 1975;8(1):33-9.).

Even if that wasn't the case, it's unclear if octopamine could cause significant fat loss in humans. In an in-vitro (test tube) study of octopamine applied to human fat cells, two different actions were seen. On the one hand, weak lipolysis (fat breakdown) was observed; on the other, insulin–like glucose uptake was also seen, due to oxidation by monoamine oxidase (MAO): an enzyme found in fat tissues. These two effects could conceivably cancel each other out, but there's no way to know without the relevant research.

What does the real world say for weight loss?

Octopamine is included with a variety of other compounds in OTC diet supplements, so it hasn't been possible to make any kind of independent judgement about it.

Will Brink's Recommendation

I am sure the reader (you reading this book right now) is getting tired of me using sentences like "there's no way to know without the relevant research" with so many of the supplements covered here. That's the reality with octopamine, as well as many others throughout the book, however. If it weren't true I wouldn't say it!

Anyhow, since it's readily metabolized in the gut, as well as easily broken down by MAO, it seems to me that—for octopamine to be effective at all—then larger doses than those currently contained in diet supplements would be needed.

Until more research is performed, in my opinion, there are other, better compounds available.

164

What is it?

Orlistat (tetrahydrolipistatin) is a prescription medication for weight loss that was approved in 2006 for OTC use by the US Food and Drug Administration. The manufacturer, GlaxoSmithKline Consumer Healthcare is marketing it under the brand name Alli.

The Skinny on Diet Supplements
Fact Vs Fiction

Orlistat

What is it supposed to do?

Orlistat is a lipase inhibitor. Lipases are pancreatic enzymes secreted into the small intestine that catalyze the breakdown of dietary fats (triglycerides) into free fatty acids and glycerol. Orlistat binds to lipases in the GI tract and inhibits fat digestion by approximately 30%. Intact triglycerides pass through the GI tract unabsorbed, and are excreted in the feces. By impairing fat digestion, Orlistat acts to create a caloric deficit.

What does the research say?

Both clinical trials conducted by the manufacturer and independent studies have made it clear that Orlistat can enhance the effects of a weight loss diet.

In one study by the manufacturer, 25% of patients taking Orlistat on a reduced calorie diet succeeded in losing more than 10% of their total body weight vs. 8% using placebo and diet alone.

In five other trials reported by the manufacturer, 2 to 5 times as many patients using Orlistat + diet lost more than 10% of their total body

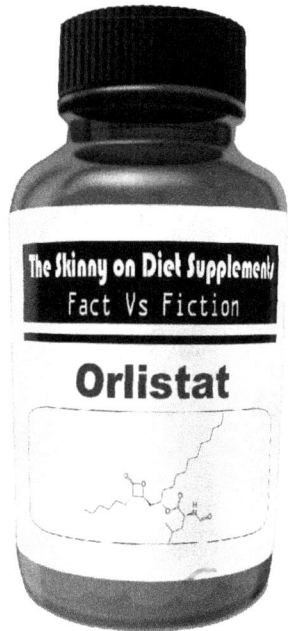

weight than patients taking a placebo + diet. The average weight loss was 13.4 lbs. for the patients on Orlistat/diet vs. 5.8 lbs. for patients on placebo/diet.

In clinical trials, improvements were also seen in levels of LDL cholesterol (avg. reduction: -4.0%), systolic and diastolic blood pressure, and glycemic control.

Positive changes have also been documented in independent studies. For example, in one recent Chinese study (*Diabet Med.* 2005 Dec;22(12):1737- 43.), Orlistat-treated patients on a mildly-reduced calorie diet achieved significantly greater weight loss than those receiving a placebo. Improvements in fasting plasma glucose, insulin sensitivity, lipid profiles and waist circumference were also noted.

Orlistat therapy may be useful for maintaining healthier blood lipid profiles as well. A small study done with 10 healthy men consuming a high fat diet demonstrated lower postprandial triacylglycerol levels, and smaller VLDL particles: a considerably less atherogenic profile than with placebo.

Orlistat has been proven effective for weight loss and clinical improvements in special populations as well. In another open study of 100 overweight patients with diabetes who were being treated through a hospital-based program, mean weight loss after 6 months was 7.1 kg. Orlistat also reduced the need for diabetes medication, irrespective of the amount of weight lost (*Curr Med Res Opin.* 2005 Nov;21(11):1885-90.).

The four-year XENDOS study also demonstrated that Orlistat therapy and lifestyle changes were more effective at reducing the incidence of Type–2 diabetes in a cohort of 3305 patients than lifestyle changes alone. Among those who completed the trial, the incidence of diabetes was 9.0% for the placebo group vs. 6.2% for the group receiving Orlistat.

The positive changes may have been due to weight loss: average weight lost was 5.8 kg in the Orlistat group vs. 3.0 kg with placebo (*Diabetes Care.* 2004 Jan;27(1):155-61.).

Orlistat plus diet therapy has also been used successfully for weight loss and psychological improvements in patients suffering from Binge Eating

166

Disorder and for improving weight loss and exercise tolerance in obese patients suffering from heart failure.

What does the real world say for weight loss?

From what I've just written, Orlistat would seem to be a pretty good bet: it helps with weight loss, and improves a variety of clinical signs of degenerative disease. And now that it's available without a prescription, could it be the fat loss miracle we've all been waiting for?

I always say, "if it seems too good to be true, it probably is," and Orlistat is no exception to that hard earned rule.

Although Orlistat has been shown to be safe in studies lasting 1-4 years, the side effects of this medication can be unpleasant.

As mentioned earlier, undigested fat is excreted. The presence of excess fat in the large intestine can lead to undesirable gastrointestinal problems: nearly 30% of Orlistat users suffer from one or more of the following symptoms:

"oily spotting from the rectum, flatus with discharge, fecal urgency, fatty/oily stool, oily evacuation, increased defecation, and fecal incontinence"

Can you say "leaky butt syndrome"?!

Furthermore, patients must adhere to a diet containing less than 30% of calories from fat, or the incidence and severity of these symptoms will increase.

In other words, taking Orlistat isn't "written permission" to indulge in high fat meals. It's quite the opposite, in fact. The side effects will increase with the fat content of a meal greatly increasing the chances of the aforementioned leaky butt syndrome (or LBS)!

In addition, Orlistat can reduce the absorption of fat-soluble nutrients: vitamins A, D, E, K, essential fatty acids, and carotenoids, making multivitamin supplementation mandatory. It may also interfere with the metabolism of other prescription medications, such as cyclosporine.

Still, some might still be willing to put up with these drawbacks, in order to take advantage of Orlistat's ability to enhance weight loss.

But is the increase in weight loss with Orlistat really that impressive?

A clue can be obtained from the product literature. The ideal patient for Orlistat treatment is someone with a BMI of 28-30 kg/m2, who

"has previously produced a weight loss of at least 2.5 kg over a period of 4 consecutive weeks."
(http://www.roche-obesity.net/xenical/xenical_spc.pdf).

In other words, Orlistat alone isn't a weight loss cure; one also has to have diet discipline and already be losing weight for it to be useful.

Independent studies have confirmed that the results from Orlistat are significant—but that's significant in a statistical sense. It doesn't mean "huge"—it just means that the losses are sufficiently different than those obtained using a placebo that it isn't likely to be due to chance or individual variation.

So how much extra weight will you lose with Orlistat? According to an independent review on Orlistat and another weight loss drug, sibutramine, the average increase in weight loss is only 2–4 kg (*Appetite.* 2006 Jan;46(1):6-10.). If you have a relatively small amount of weight to lose, this can be an advantage, but is a negligible amount if you have a lot of weight to lose.

In addition, other interventions have been shown to be just as good—if not better—than using Orlistat. A small study (*Public Health.* 2006 Jan;120(1):76-82.) compared the use of short-term Orlistat + diet vs. aerobic exercise training + diet.

The researchers found similar amounts of weight were lost, but the exercise group lost more total fat, and increased their cardiopulmonary fitness as well.

Another, larger study on weight regain in women who lost weight using a very low energy liquid diet (VLED) found that the group receiving meal replacements during a 1-year weight maintenance program maintained their weight loss just as well as the group receiving Orlistat.

168

The researchers concluded that:

"meal replacements may be a viable alternative strategy to medications for weight maintenance"

(*J Am Coll Nutr.* 2005 Oct;24(5):347-53.).

Will Brink's Recommendation

I personally believe that the drawbacks of this drug outweigh the benefits, particularly since alternatives can produce results that are at least as good. If you wish to try Orlistat, however, be sure to follow the manufacturer's instructions to the letter to optimize your results and limit unpleasant side effects.

The recommended dose of prescription strength Orlistat is 120 mg to be taken 3 times a day, just before, with, or up to 1 hour after a meal containing some fat. The diet should contain no more than 30% of total calories from fat, and the fat should be evenly distributed over the three meals that Orlistat is taken with.

The bottom line here is I inherently dislike any drug or supplement that works by blocking the uptake of macronutrients, (i.e., carbs, proteins, and fats) and Orlistat confirms why.

Possible side effects and drug interactions

- Patients should not use alli if they have had an organ transplant or if they are taking medicine to reduce organ rejection

- Patients should not use alli if taking cyclosporine; alli can reduce levels of cyclosporine in the blood

- Patients on warfarin should be advised to talk with their doctor before taking alli; they will need to be monitored closely for changes in coagulation parameters and have their blood tested regularly, which is standard for any individual taking warfarin who is considering starting a new concomitant drug

- Patients taking medicine for thyroid disease should be advised to talk to their doctor before taking alli

- alli does not negatively interfere with diabetes medication; in fact, a clinical trial has demonstrated that patients taking orlistat have been able to reduce or discontinue their diabetes medicine[1]

- No clinically relevant drug interactions were seen when alli was taken in combination with weight loss drugs, such as phentermine or sibutramine[2]

- Patients should stop use and ask their doctor if they develop itching, yellow eyes or skin, dark urine or loss of appetite. There have been rare reports of liver injury in people taking orlistat.

More important usage information

- A multivitamin containing vitamins A, D, E, K, and beta-carotene once daily at bedtime is recommended. Orlistat inhibits 25% of dietary fat, and may reduce the absorption of some fat-soluble vitamins. alli and a multivitamin should not be taken at the same time to gain the most benefit of a multivitamin. However, if they are taken at the same time, at least 70% of the fat-soluble vitamins would be absorbed

- Do not use if pregnant or breastfeeding

- Do not use if an individual has been diagnosed with problems absorbing food or is allergic to any of the ingredients in an alli capsule

- Do not use if BMI < 25

- Individuals should be advised to talk with their doctor before using alli if they have had gall bladder problems, kidney stones, pancreatitis or if severe abdominal pain occurs

Source:
http://www.allihcp.com/IntroAlli_DrugInteractions.aspx

PEPTIDE FM

What is it?

Peptide FM, also known as globin digest, is made from certain proteins treated with proteases (enzymes) to create peptides (oligopeptides) of a specific length and sequence. Peptide FM is derived from various proteins, including cow's blood (yuk).

What is it suppose to do?

Peptide FM is supposed to be able to reduce fat deposition from both the intake of fat and carbohydrates in the diet at both the digestive and cellular level. In theory, Peptide FM inhibits lipogenesis (fat storage) in both liver and adipose (fat) tissue as well as inhibiting certain enzymes involved with the production and subsequent storage of fat in fat cells.

An increase in beta–oxidation (fat burning) and a reduction of triglycerides, along with other benefits are claimed.

What does the research say?

Peptide FM appears to have some interesting properties that may be of use to people trying to lose weight. In-vitro (test tube) and animal research suggests Peptide FM works on a variety of mechanisms to prevent the absorption of dietary fats and synthesis of body fat.

Its effects can be found at both the digestive and cellular levels. On the digestive level, Peptide FM was shown to reduce the uptake of fats and carbohydrates by mechanisms yet to be fully explained. On the cellular level, it was found to increase beta-oxidation (fat burning) and inhibit certain enzymes involved with the storage of fat (FAS and GPDH) and the production of triglycerides.

In mice, rats, pigs, and dogs, Peptide FM was shown to reduce body fat and reduce serum triglycerides from eating both fats and carbohydrates.

In a double-blind clinical trial using real live human beings, Peptide FM reduced body fat by approximately 3% in one month in people taking about 1.6 g a day. In this study, doses ranged from about 0.6 g/day (600 mg a day) to 2 g/day (2000 mg per day). They concluded that the higher dose was more effective than the lower dose.

So what's the downside of Peptide FM research?

For one thing, exactly how it does what it does is not well understood, but it does not appear to pose any dangers to the user. It may work by mimicking some of the satiety hormones such as CCK (see section on glyomacropeptide for more info on CCK) or by causing a release of those hormones. There may be direct effects from Peptide FM on preventing fat synthesis as mentioned above.

The real problem with the studies mentioned is they have never seen the light of day in a peer reviewed medical or scientific journal.

Most of the information we have on Peptide FM, including the information above, comes from "in house" research published by the Japanese pharmaceutical company that manufactures it. There are however, a few studies that were published in 1996 and 1998 on Peptide FM regarding its effects on blood lipid levels (i.e. cholesterol and triglycerides.).

A 1998 study called "**Suppressive Effect of Globin Digest on Postprandial Hyperlipidemia in Male Volunteers**" came to some interesting conclusions. The study was a parallel crossover trial conducted with men who consumed a high fat diet (25 g fat, 7.6 g carbohydrate, 1.9 g protein and 0.7 g sodium chloride) or the same diet supplemented with Peptide FM. The amounts used in the study ranged from 1 to 4 grams of Peptide FM per day.

In the men receiving the higher doses of Peptide FM, blood levels of triglycerides were greatly reduced.

The researchers concluded:

"In these trials, globin digest (Peptide FM) reduced the increase in serum chylomicron triglyceride concentrations as a result of the ingestion of a high fat diet. This hypotriglyceridemic effect of globin digest may be valuable for preventing obesity and in lowering the incidence of cardiovascular diseases."

Another study found essentially the same thing after feeding people olive oil. This study also looked at some of the possible mechanisms through which Peptide FM achieved these impressive results. The study found Peptide FM did not suppress peristaltic movement nor delay gastric emptying, that is, Peptide FM did not change the rate at which food was moved through the digestive tract, but did find that the excretion of the olive oil was greater than that of the control group.

More importantly to weight loss perhaps, the study found Peptide FM caused an activation of certain enzymes involved in fat metabolism and clearance (hepatic triglyceride lipase, or HTGL). The study concluded that Peptide FM inhibited fat absorption in the digestive tract and enhanced activity of certain enzymes involved in clearance of dietary fats. These results could have an effect on weight loss.

What does the real world say for weight loss?

Very few people have used Peptide FM in the U.S., so feedback in this country has been limited so far. I can not offer you a clear picture of its real world effectiveness at this time. It's been 6 years since the first version of this book, and feedback is pretty much non-existent.

Will Brink's Recommendation

It is my understanding that Peptide FM has been sold in Japan for some time as a weight loss product. If this product proves to be as good as its claim and research suggests, it may be a useful addition to the dieter's arsenal of fat loss nutrients.

The studies I have read make it seem almost too good to be true, and things that appear too good to be true, usually means the catch hasn't been discovered. For example, studies indicate that although Peptide FM

173

can block the absorption of dietary fats and carbohydrates, it does not interfere with the absorption of fat soluble vitamins and essential fatty acids.

Sorry, but the human body rarely, if ever, works on the "having your cake and eating it too" principle.

There are a few companies in the U.S. that sell Peptide FM as a dietary supplement, but it is not a popular item in the U.S. yet. Peptide FM is also quite expensive and using the 1-4 grams per day needed is a costly proposition. No side effects have been reported in any of the studies.

Peptide FM comes under the "might be a worth a try" category if the person does not mind parting with the money.

Peptide FM looked modestly promising in the studies done, but perhaps due to cost or poor marketing, or lack luster feedback, it never caught on as a weight loss product. Currently, I don't know of any companies currently selling it.

PHASEOLUS VULGARIS EXTRACT

What is it?

Phaseolus vulgaris extract (PVE) is considered a "starch blocker" supplement and is derived from white kidney beans.

What is it supposed to do?

The extract from white kidney beans (Phaseolus vulgaris) contains an alpha–amylase inhibitor. Alpha-amylase is a digestive enzyme that breaks down starches. In theory, taking phaseolus extracts would inhibit the digestion and absorption of carbohydrates.

Sellers of PVE (and other starch blockers) tell people things like "you can eat all the starches you want and not gain weight" and other claims that smack of the too-good-to-be-true syndrome.

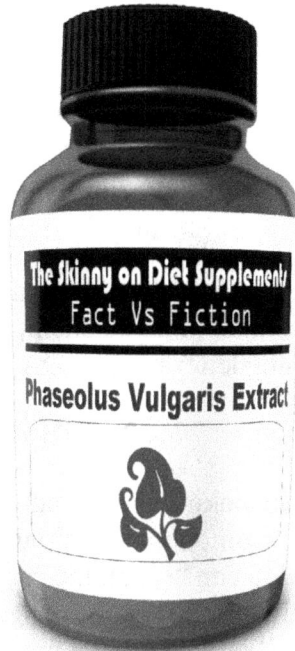

What does the research say?

In general, studies looking at PVE and weight loss are underwhelming to say the least. They either find no weight loss (*Hum Nutr Clin Nutr*. 1983 Jul;37(4):301-5, *N Engl J Med*. 1982 Dec 2;307(23):1413-6., *Science*. 1983 Jan 28;219(4583):393-5) or very slight weight loss. One study already referenced above stated:

"We conclude that starch-blocker tablets do not inhibit the digestion and absorption of starch calories in human beings."

The one study that did find some positive results (*Altern Med Rev*. 2004 Mar;9(1):63-9) found the group getting the supplement lost 3.79 lbs. vs.

1.65 lbs. for placebo, over a period of 8 weeks, which did not reach statistical significance. Not very impressive to say the least...PVE may also be potentially dangerous as studies suggest it may cause deficiencies in other nutrients (*J Nutr.* 1995 Jun;125(6):1554-62, *Plant Foods Hum Nutr.* 1992 Apr;42(2):135-42), and has been found to retard growth in animals.

What does the real world say for weight loss?

In general, people that have used PVE have reported no weight loss.

Will Brink's Recommendation

I don't think it will take a rocket scientist to figure out I am going to give this supplement a big thumbs down. In fact, the manufacturer of the US supplement, Pharmachem, a major manufacturer of PVE, was sent a warning letter by the FDA

(http://www.fda.gov/foi/warning_letters/g5083d.htm)

to stop making unsubstantiated claims for fat loss on their web site and other promotional materials. The often pushed claim by sellers of PVE that you can "eat all the carbs you want..." is complete rubbish, to put it mildly. It may also be dangerous. I also dislike any supplement that works by blocking the uptake of a major nutrient (in this case carbohydrates), which invariably leads to potential problems.

If a person needs such a supplement, then they are simply eating too many carbohydrates in the first place!

PHOSPHATIDYLSERINE

What is it?

Phosphatidylserine (PS) is a phospholipid found in the human body with particularly high concentrations in the brain and nervous system.

What's it supposed to do?

Phosphatidylserine (PS) is supplement that holds great promise for people suffering from various pathologies that affect the brain, such as certain forms of dementia, Alzheimer's, and others. Early European studies showed that phosphatidylserine could slow and reverse the rate of brain cell aging in laboratory animals.

PS also restored mental function in older animals to levels exceeding those found in some younger animals (Although studies in humans with Alzheimer's disease were less impressive, PS still produced improvements in cognitive function).

Research has shown that in addition to improving neural function, PS appears to enhance energy metabolism in brain cells. In the brain, PS helps maintain cell membrane integrity and may protect brain cells against the functional deterioration that occurs with "normal" aging. PS is usually derived from soy.

There is controversy over whether or not soy-based PS is as effective as it's not identical to the PS used in most studies that were derived from cow's brains.

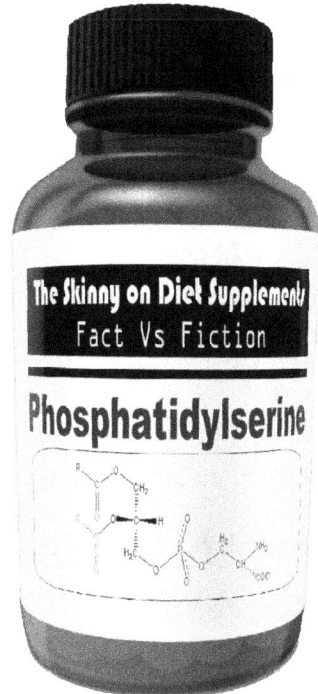

Brain tissue has been found to be especially rich in PS and it appears aging causes a decline in the PS content of cells throughout the body. So, it's no wonder that longevity groups and individuals concerned with brain function due to various causes have taken an interest in PS.

One effect of PS may be its ability to reduce levels of the catabolic (muscle wasting) hormone cortisol after exercise. Two early studies done in Italy appeared to show that chronic intakes of PS reduced the release of cortisol after intense exercise.

When the body senses stress, whether physical and/or emotional, it releases cortisol as part of the "fight or flight" cascade that prepares us for short term survival. Prolonged stress from malnutrition,surgery, overtraining, and sleep deprivation, as well as psychological stress, causes a systemic effect that includes increased cortisol secretion. This causes a decline in certain aspects of immune system and other problems.

So as you can see, over long periods of time, high cortisol levels are detrimental to our overall health and muscle mass.

What does PS offer the dieter in particular?

Recent studies suggest that the hormone cortisol is also associated with abdominal fat. This has lead to a bunch of "cortisol control" type formulas, most of which will contain some PS due to the association of high cortisol levels and abdominal fat.

What does the research have to say?

Research looking at PS for weight loss specifically is lacking.

What does the real world say for weight loss?

No one has reported weight loss from the addition of PS to their diet and supplement regimen.

Will Brink's Recommendation.

PS does suffer from one key drawback, which is its sheer cost. The study that found PS reduced post-exercise cortisol levels the most, used 800 mg per day with 10 well-trained subjects who were intentionally over-trained, and found approximately a 20% reduction in post-exercise cortisol levels.

The study also found post-workout soreness reduced and general feelings of 'well being' increased in the group using PS. At the 800 mg doses used, it's an expensive proposition, but possibly worth the cost. However, the original studies out of Italy found PS lowered cortisol used only 50 and 75 mg per day, so this may at least be a starting dose to try, though I seriously doubt that dose would be effective.

For general health and other uses as mentioned above, PS looks worth using.

For weight loss, there is no real proof it will reduce either abdominal fat or whole body fat. Marketers of cortisol control formulas (as usual) far overstate the effects of their products and far more research has to occur with PS looking at weight loss to bother spending the money. It's also essential to know these formulas on the market never contain the needed doses used in the research, so don't bother with them.

If someone wants to use PS, buy PS only and try a starting dose of at least 100 mg 3 times per day and move up to 300 mg 3 times per day.

PS gets a big "thumbs up" as a general health supplement. As a weight loss supplement, however, I can't recommend it at this time.

Possible side effects and drug interactions

Moderate Interaction Be cautious with this combination

Drying medications (Anticholinergic drugs) interacts with PHOSPHATIDYLSERINE

Some drying medications are called anticholinergic drugs. Phosphatidylserine might increase chemicals that can decrease the effects of these drying medications.

179

Some drying medications include atropine, scopolamine, and some medications used for allergies (antihistamines) and for depression (antidepressants).

Medications for Alzheimer's disease (Acetylcholinesterase (AChE) inhibitors) interacts with PHOSPHATIDYLSERINE

Phosphatidylserine might increase a chemical in the body called acetylcholine. Medications for Alzheimer's disease called acetylcholinesterase inhibitors also increase the chemical acetylcholine. Taking phosphatidylserine along with medications for Alzheimer's disease might increase effects and side effects of medications for Alzheimer's disease.

Some acetylcholinesterase medications include donepezil (Aricept), tacrine (Cognex), rivastigmine (Exelon), and galantamine (Reminyl, Razadyne).

Various medications used for glaucoma, Alzheimer's disease, and other conditions (Cholinergic drugs) interacts with PHOSPHATIDYLSERINE

Phosphatidylserine might increase a chemical in the body called acetylcholine. This chemical is similar to some medications used for glaucoma, Alzheimer's disease, and other conditions. Taking phosphatidylserine with these medications might increase the chance of side effects.

Some of these medications used for glaucoma, Alzheimer's disease, and other conditions include pilocarpine (Pilocar and others), and others.

Source: WebMD
http://www.webmd.com/vitamins-supplements/ingredientmono-992-PHOSPHATIDYLSERINE.aspx?activeIngredientId=992&activeIngredientName=PHOSPHATIDYLSERINE

PIPERINE (BIOPERINE™)

What is it?

Piperine is the alkaloid in black pepper (Piper nigrum L) responsible for its pungent, "peppery" taste. Bioperine™ is a commercial black pepper extract that has been standardized to 95% piperine.

Bioperine™ is the form of piperine found in most OTC diet supplements.

What is it supposed to do?

Although it has other biological activities, piperine is included in supplements to enhance the absorption of other nutrients. It's not a weight loss supplement in the literal sense but pops up in various weight loss formulas.

What does the research say?

Piperine is a vanilloid receptor agonist (*Br J Pharmacol*. 2005 Mar;144(6):781- 90.). Vanilloid receptors are involved in the perception of pain and inflammation. Capsaicin—the compound that gives chili peppers their heat—is also a vanilloid receptor agonist. Translated, it stimulates the receptor and thus why your mouth burns like crazy when eating hot chili peppers and why criminals on the Fox show "Cops" fall to the ground when hit in the face with pepper spray….but I digress…..

In animal experiments, co-administration of piperine increases the absorption of drugs or nutrients such as EGCG from green tea (*J Nutr*. 2004 Aug;134(8):1948-52.), beta–lactam antibiotics (*Indian J Exp Biol*.

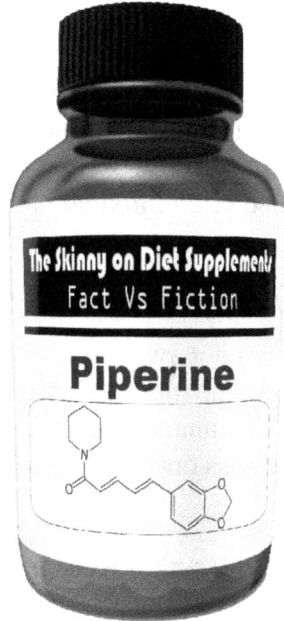

2002 Mar;40(3):277-81.), and curcumin (*Planta Med.* 1998 May;64(4):353-6.).

In experiments with human volunteers, piperine increased the absorption of coenzyme Q10 , as well as beta-carotene. Sabinsa Corporation, the manufacturer of Bioperine™ claims increased absorption for selenium, Vitamin B6, and Vitamin C with Bioperine™ as well, although complete data is not given.

In rats and mice, piperine is known to delay gastric emptying and inhibit gastrointestinal transit (*Planta Med.* 2001 Mar;67(2):176-9.). This almost certainly plays a role in enhancing nutrient absorption. Piperine also has antioxidant activity and even has potential as an antidepressant.

What does the real world say for weight loss?

I am not aware of any commercial diet supplements that have magically become more effective with the addition of piperine. In theory, it could help enhance the absorption of useful compounds, but will not make useless ones effective!

Will Brink's Recommendation

Most of the human studies on nutrient absorption have used a dose of 5 mg piperine. While a lower dose may also be effective, there is no information available to confirm this.

It's difficult to give any relevant advice concerning supplements containing piperine. It is a potentially useful addition, but any supplement including it should be judged by the other ingredients present. Studies comparing one weight loss formula or ingredient containing piperine vs. the same without piperine to see if it actually would enhance the effects of said formula/ingredient are lacking.

So at best all that can be said is, in theory, the addition of piperine to a weight loss may enhance absorption but it's unclear what effects that will have at this time. If you see it in a formula, don't worry about it.

PYRUVATE

What is it?

Pyruvate is technically a byproduct of glucose (blood sugar) metabolism. When the body breaks down glucose for energy it enters what is called the glycolytic pathway. Glucose enters the glycolytic pathway and is broken down through successive enzymatic steps arriving at pyruvate.

Think of pyruvate as half a glucose molecule, or glucose divided into two; that's basically what it is. Once pyruvate is formed it can enter the all important TCA cycle, which is the ultimate producer of ATP and other high energy compounds in the body.

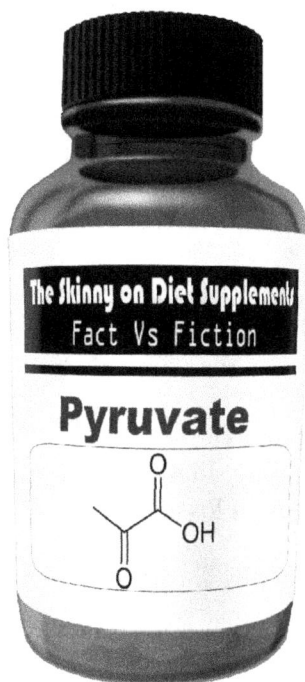

The Skinny on Diet Supplements
Fact Vs Fiction

Pyruvate

What is it supposed to do?

The various companies selling pyruvate claim it will increase energy, improve athletic performance, and help people trying to lose weight get more "bang for the buck" from their diets.

What does the research say?

The human studies done with pyruvate have looked promising but not miraculous for weight loss. The majority of research on pyruvate and weight loss has been carried out at the University of Pittsburgh by a Dr. Stanko and colleagues.

One study took two groups of obese women who were put on very low calorie diets (VLCD) for 21 days. One group had approximately 20% of their low calorie diets replaced with pyruvate and they lost more weight overall (5.9 kg vs. 4.3 kg) and fat in particular (4.0 kg vs. 2.7 kg) than the group that did not receive the pyruvate.

An earlier study done by the same group of researchers had similar results with basically the same setup (i.e. very low calorie/low-fat diets and pyruvate replacing roughly 20% of the study participants' calories).

In one of the most recent studies done by Dr. Stanko and colleagues, 17 women were put on extremely low calorie diets for three weeks followed by diets consisting of 150% of maintenance calories to see if pyruvate and dihydroxyacetone (another three carbon metabolite of glucose) could partially block the rebound weight gained from such low calorie diets.

The group that received the pyruvate and dihydroxyacetone while eating the high calorie part of the study gained less weight (+1.8 kg vs +2.9 kg) than the women who did not receive these glucose metabolites.

In one of these studies, the women getting the pyruvate sustained a slightly higher metabolic rate, which is also important for long term weight loss.

Finally, for preventing weight gain, one study found that on a 46% fat diet (that's a high fat diet) pyruvate failed to prevent weight gain but it did slightly reduce total cholesterol and diastolic blood pressure, therefore appearing to have some health benefits for the people eating a high fat diet.

Research appeared to show that a dose as low as 6 grams per day caused statistically significant weight loss, with an increase in lean body mass (muscle).

It was a small study, however, and other research generally indicates a need for much higher intakes to get a response from pyruvate.

Pyruvate may have some potential use in the treatment and control of Type–2 diabetes and other ailments. Diabetes is characterized as a disease relating to abnormalities in blood sugar regulation. Research was conducted to see what effect pyruvate might have on blood sugar levels and utilization.

184

The main job of the hormone insulin is to pull glucose out of the blood stream and deposit it into other compartments such as muscle tissue (to be stored as glycogen for future energy needs). When food intake exceeds glycogen storage capacity, the body can convert glucose into body fat.

In Type–2 diabetes the main problem is "insulin resistance." That is, tissues have become unable to accept blood sugar from insulin with the result of the blood sugar building up in the blood stream causing a host of physical problems common to Type–2 diabetics (see discussion on Syndrome X in the section on chromium for more information on blood sugar related health issues).

Since skeletal muscles are the main repository for glucose following a meal, it is easy to see that anything that improves the muscles' ability to react to insulin (i.e. improve insulin sensitivity) will help the Type–2 diabetic control this disease.

One study using pyruvate with Type–2 diabetics showed reductions in blood glucose and possible improvements in insulin sensitivity. If future research shows similar results with pyruvate and diabetics, it could have legitimate uses in diseases involving blood sugar regulation, though further research is clearly indicated.

Some research points to possible performance applications of pyruvate. As mentioned previously, pyruvate can be thought of as half a glucose molecule, which is to say that glucose is a six carbon molecule and pyruvate is a three carbon compound derived from glucose. The body stores glucose in the muscles for future energy needs in the form of glycogen: when we exercise, the body breaks down this stored energy or "muscle sugar" to fuel the production of ATP for energy.

It should come as no real surprise that the intake of pyruvate can spare muscle glycogen during exercise and increase the rate of glycogen storage in the muscles after exercise.

For runners and other endurance athletes, this could result in greater endurance. There has been research demonstrating pyruvate improved leg exercise endurance and improved endurance on a group of people tested on an arm crank machine. An increase in stored muscle glycogen causes the muscles cells to swell, thus making the muscles appear larger. Pyruvate may have uses for bodybuilders as well as endurance athletes.

The practice of "carb loading" to increase glycogen stores and make the muscles appear larger is a common practice of bodybuilders pre-contest and pyruvate might also have uses during a carb loading phase, although I see no advantages over eating good old carbohydrates for the same purpose.

What does the real world say for weight loss?

The bulk of feedback I have gotten regarding pyruvate has been negative regarding weight loss. This may be due to the fact that no one can afford to take the dose needed for an effect on weight loss. Or it could be the possibility that pyruvate simply does not affect weight loss. The form pyruvate comes in could also be an issue.

Will Brink's Recommendation

So what are the potential downsides of pyruvate? With only exception, all the research to date has been based on very high doses of pyruvate. For example, in the study that showed pyruvate reduced weight gain with VLCDs, 15 grams of pyruvate plus 75 grams of dihydroxyacetone were used.

In the various studies that showed pyruvate assisted in weight loss on very low to moderate calorie intakes, doses ranged from 30 to 53 grams, with pyruvate making up 20% of total calories. That's a heck of a lot of pyruvate. A person would have to take 60 x 500 milligram capsules a day to get the 30 grams of pyruvate that was used in the research!

The improvements demonstrated in exercise performance and endurance used at least 20 grams which would equal 40 x 500 milligram capsules daily. Besides the obvious inconvenience of taking this many capsules, the costs would be prohibitive.

Finally, the amount of weight lost by the group getting pyruvate was not so significantly different from the people not getting the supplement to warrant the investment.

Another important issue is the form pyruvate comes in. Currently, pyruvate offered as either sodium (sodium pyruvate) or calcium (calcium pyruvate) salts. The intake of 15 grams of sodium pyruvate will add 3 grams (3000 milligrams) of sodium to a person's diet.

Thus, the intake of these forms of pyruvate may be limited by the amount of sodium and/or calcium a person wants in their diet or is safe to add to the diet. High intakes of either could potentially cause mineral imbalances over the long term.

There are other variations of pyruvate that would prevent this problem, such as pyruvate connected to the amino acid glycine to make pyruvylglycine. This form would eliminate the dangers of mineral imbalances but has not been well tested in people and is even more expensive than the two types currently being marketed!

Several companies marketing pyruvate and a few magazine articles have claimed that 5 grams might be as effective as the much higher amounts used in the research. This information is based on extrapolations from animal research but there is little human data that shows this to be true.

Therefore, I would not get all that excited regarding those claims that 5 grams will work as well as the higher doses or will "prime the energy pump" to quote one marketing document. It is possible that pyruvate could end up being a useful part of the dieter's arsenal, but the jury is still out as to exactly how useful it will be, exactly how it works, what are the exact doses needed, and for how long it needs to be taken.

So far, I have met very few people who felt they lost weight using pyruvate. There have been no serious side effects reported, nor would I expect any.

People interested in using pyruvate should take at least 6 grams (6000 milligrams) per day as a minimum amount, assuming the one study that found that 6 grams a day to be effective, is correct. I assume I don't have to repeat that weight loss formulas containing a few hundred milligrams of pyruvate are 100% worthless, right? Hope not...

Other names for Pyruvate

Acetylformic Acid

Alpha-Keto Acid

Alpha-Ketopropionic Acid

Calcium Pyruvate

Calcium Pyruvate Monohydrate

Creatine Pyruvate

Magnesium Pyruvate

2-Oxopropanoate, 2-Oxypropanoic Acid

Piruvato

Potassium Pyruvate

Proacemic Acid

Pyruvic Acid

Sodium Pyruvate

SALVIA SCLAREA (SCLAREOLIDE)

What is it?

Salvia sclarea is also known as "Clary Sage": a medicinal herb used today as an essential oil and for aromatherapy. Extracts of clary sage flowers and leaves are used in the food and cosmetic industries, as a fragrance and flavor additive. In recent years, a semi-synthetic compound derived from clary sage, sclareolide, has been included in several OTC fat loss supplements, due to its alleged thermogenic properties.

What is it supposed to do?

Sclareolide is claimed to be an activator of adenylate cyclase, the enzyme that catalyzes the production of cyclic AMP (cAMP). cAMP is a cellular "second messenger" needed for the activation of another enzyme, hormone-sensitive lipase (HSL), which catalyzes the breakdown of stored body fat. See also my comments on forskolin which works through essentially the same mechanism.

What does the research say?

There is virtually no research available to support the claims made for sclareolide or extracts of Salvia sclarea for fat loss. The makers of one diet supplement cite an unpublished report produced by a commercial laboratory (*Anonymous*, Sclareolide Effect on cAMP in Two Cell Lines. Unpublished report by *NovaScreen*. 2003; 19 pp.). There is also a single

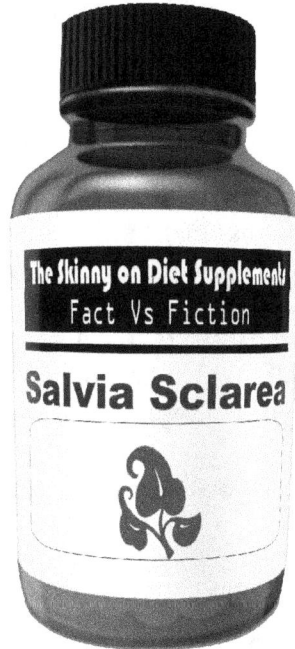

published study in Bulgarian that demonstrated an increase in cAMP in cultured brain tissues from rats exposed to "sclareol glycol."

That's it! How does one come to recommend this supplement for weight loss based on the above? Beats the heck out of me….Never has so much been made from so little. Didn't Winston Churchill say that? Never mind….

It may be that individual companies may have conducted internal research. If so, they've been very shy about revealing their data, preferring instead to rely on unsubstantiated claims for efficacy, and that NEVER bodes well for a product.

Assuming that the in-vitro (test tube) studies show a genuine effect, would that make supplements containing sclareolide effective fat burners? Not necessarily.

Direct exposure to cells in culture can produce different effects than something that has to pass through the digestive system first. In addition, there is the dose to consider. Compounds applied directly to cells can't give you any valid information about how much of a compound needs to be given to a person or animal to have similar effects.

What does the real world say for weight loss?

Not much—there's very little to say. Supplements containing sclareolide also contain a number of other ingredients, which make it impossible to form any independent judgment on its effectiveness.

Will Brink's Recommendation

Sclareolide is listed as GRAS* by the FDA for use in foods, cosmetics and tobacco. It appears to be reasonably safe at the doses given in most OTC supplements, but in reality, research is lacking. Due to the lack of credible human or animal studies, I cannot recommend this ingredient at this time for weight loss.

* = Generally Recognized as Safe

SESAMIN

What is it?

Sesamin is a naturally occurring lignan extracted from sesame seeds. Plant lignans can be converted in the human body to the mammalian lignans enterodiol and enterolactone: compounds that mimic some of the effects of estrogens. Mammalian lignans have been shown to exert protective effects against hormone dependent cancers.

What is it supposed to do?

Sesamin increases mitochondrial oxidation of fatty acids in the liver and muscle, which—ideally—increases the amount fat burning. It simultaneously reduces levels of lipogenic (fat storing) enzymes and increases serum levels of vitamin E.

What does the research say?

In animal studies, sesamin inhibits the degradation of gamma–tocopherol (a form of vitamin E) which increases the amount detectable in tissue and plasma This effect protects against in-vivo peroxidation of essential fatty acids (*J Nutr Sci Vitaminol* (Tokyo). 2003 Aug;49(4):270-6.). Sesamin also has anti-inflammatory effects in rats. Sesamin-enriched diets reduced conversion of omega–6 fatty acids to pro-inflammatory arachidonic acid and augmented the anti-inflammatory effects of omega–3 fatty acids from flax oil (*Am J Clin Nutr*. 2000 Sep;72(3):804-8.).

Rats fed sesamin-enriched diets showed increased hepatic fatty acid oxidation, which was elevated even more when combined with fish oil

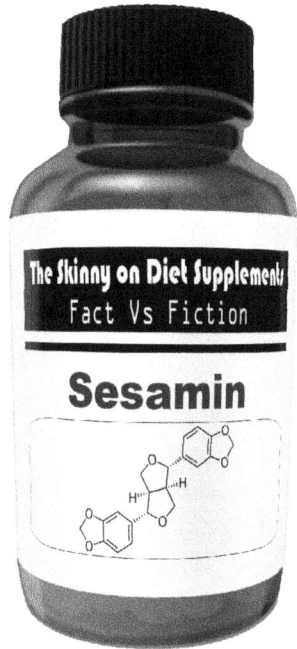

(*Biochim Biophys Acta*. 2004 Jun 1;1682(1-3):80-91.). Fatty acid synthesis was also reduced by sesamin. These effects were attenuated, however, in mice and hamsters.

Feeding studies correlated with in-vitro data demonstrate that sesamin is converted to enterolactone in humans. Consumption of sesame seed or oil muffins containing sesamin increased serum vitamin E in humans (*Nutr Cancer*. 2001;39(1):66-71.).

What does the real world say for weight loss?

User feedback has been very mixed for sesamin, with some reporting positive—but not dramatic—results, while others report no fat loss at all. Some feel that it's been more helpful in reducing fat gains when bulking than for actual fat loss.

Will Brink's Recommendation

There appear to be health benefits to using sesamin, although data on fat loss in animals and humans is lacking. Bottom line is, until more information is available, I feel that there are better fat loss options available, but it won't do you any harm if you want to give the stuff a try.

TETRADECYLTHIOACETIC ACID

What is it?

Tetradecylthioacetic acid (TTA) is known as a "3–thia substituted fatty acid"— a sulfur atom has been substituted for the third carbon atom in the fatty acid chain, making it a fatty acid analog.

What is it supposed to do?

TTA is a "peroxisome proliferator activated receptor alpha" (PPAR–alpha) agonist. PPAR–alpha is one of a family of mitochondrial receptors and is involved in the regulation of beta–oxidation, which is the process of burning fat for energy. PPAR–alpha activation increases the expression of the enzymes involved in fatty acid oxidation. The increased enzyme activity is supposed to amplify fat burning.

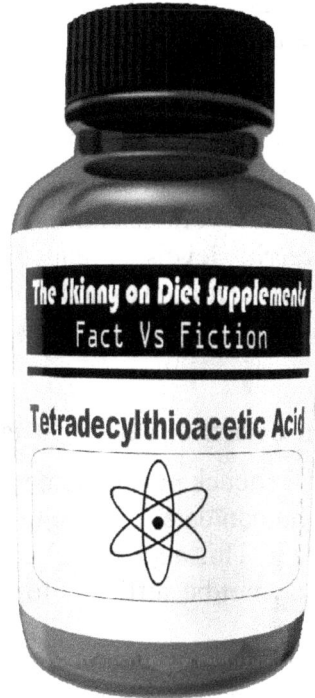

What does the research say?

Cell culture studies have demonstrated TTA is able to stimulate the growth of mitochondria in skeletal muscle fibers and increase the expression of carnitine palmitoyltransferase and fatty acyl–CoA oxidase (*Biol Cell*. 2000 Aug;92(5):317-29.) which are two key enzymes involved in beta-oxidation.

Other in-vitro research suggests that it has antioxidant activity, reduces the formation of triglycerdes, and has anti-tumor activity. Studies in animals confirm that it can reduce cholesterol levels, inhibit LDL ("bad" cholesterol) oxidation, and lower serum triglycerides.

There is a single study in rats that shows fat loss effects. The study, **"Tetradecylthioacetic acid prevents high fat diet induced adiposity and insulin resistance"** (*J Lipid Res.* 2002 May;43(5):742-50.), demonstrated that 150–300 mg/kg/day TTA increased insulin sensitivity and reduced fat gains in genetically obese Zucker rats given a high fat diet.

There is also a study in humans undergoing anti-retroviral therapy for HIV. One gram of TTA/day combined with a cholesterol-lowering diet produced favorable changes in cholesterol levels, HDL/LDL ratios, and triglyceride levels. A reduction in tumor necrosis factor alpha-a marker of inflammation was also noted. No weight or body composition changes were reported, however.

What does the real world say for weight loss?

User feedback on supplements containing TTA has been mixed. The only human data we have to go on is the study on HIV patients, who took 1 g. This appears to be a therapeutic dose for reducing blood lipids, but may not be sufficient to see fat loss effects—if there are any.

Most of the supplements available contain less than this. The study on obese mice used doses of 150 mg/kg/day: the equivalent dose for a 100 kg human would be 15 grams!

Needless to state, it wouldn't be practical or cost-effective to try to get a dose this large from the supplements currently on the market. In addition, there's no information on TTA's safety or the effects of long term use.

Will Brink's Recommendation

TTA is an interesting compound that appears to have positive effects on blood lipids and inflammation in doses available in certain supplements. So for overall health and well-being, it gets a tentative "thumbs up" from me. For fat loss, however, I have to give it a "thumbs down" at this time: there's simply not enough information to go on.

194

THYROMIMETICS

What are they?

"Thyromimetics" are metabolites of the active thyroid hormone triiodothyronine (T3), which may have biological activity that overlaps that of the parent compound.

What are they supposed to do?

Thyromimetics are alleged to increase basal metabolic rate similar to T3 and promote fat burning.

What does the research say?

There are several different thyroid hormone analogs in OTC diet supplements, that are known by acronyms: "DIAC" (diiodothyroacetic acid), "Triprop," (3,5,3'-triiodothyropropionic acid), and "Diprop" (3,5-diiodothryropropionic acid). Another, known as "TRIAC" (triiodothryroacetic acid) was determined by the FDA to be an "unapproved new drug."

Supplements containing TRIAC (a.k.a. "Tiratricol") were recalled by the FDA and withdrawn from the market. Tiratricol is known to cause symptoms of both hyperthyroidism and hypothyroidism, due to suppression of thyroid stimulating hormone, which is needed for normal thyroid hormone release.

The take home message is that there are potential risks associated with taking thyroid hormone analogs. Different metabolites have different effects, so it's difficult to make predictions about how the effects of different metabolites ingested in larger-than-normal amounts.

It is interesting to note that, although TRIAC obviously has physiological effects and was marketed as a weight loss ingredient, no actual effects on weight loss were found in a study of overweight adults

195

on a 1200 kcal/ day diet. Subjects receiving 2.8 mg/day TRIAC for 2 months lost no more weight than controls on the diet alone; nor were there any significant differences in blood lipid improvements. The case reports on side effects noted above used doses between 3 and 6 mg/day, so it's safe to say that—while an increased dose might be more effective for fat loss—the risk of side effects outweighs any potential benefits.

What about compounds like DIAC, Triprop and Diprop?

There's very little data to work with for DIAC and Triprop. Most of the studies done on these compounds are cell culture studies designed to look at receptor binding affinities, and offer little practical information we can use to make judgments.

Diprop (a.k.a. "DITPA") is being researched as a possible therapy for congestive heart failure: it can strengthen the heart without increasing heart rate and metabolic rate (Thyroid. 2002 Jun;12(6):527-33.). That's promising news for patients, but disappointing news for anyone thinking this compound might substantially increase metabolic rate. As a therapy for heart failure, diprop looks very promising, but for fat loss, it's likely to be a dud.

What does the real world say for weight loss?

One supplement containing DIAC has gotten generally favorable reviews, although users are taking twice the maximum recommended dose to achieve results. At that level, hot flashes, lethargy, and some rebound weight gain have also been reported.

I have not heard any feedback—good or bad—on supplements containing Diprop or Triprop.

Will Brink's Recommendation

I am hesitant, to say the least, to recommend any product with the potential to affect normal thyroid output. In one of the case reports of Tiratricol-induced hypothyroidism, it took nearly 5 months for normal thyroid function to be completely regained.

In my opinion, taking thyromimetic compounds is playing with fire; if they don't work, they're a ripoff, and if they do, then the risk of side effects is high. There are better and safer options available.

Possible Drug Interactions to be aware of

Major Interaction Do not take this combination

Stimulant drugs interacts with TIRATRICOL

Stimulant drugs speed up the nervous system. By speeding up the nervous system, stimulant medications can make you feel jittery and speed up your heartbeat. Tiratricol might also speed up the nervous system. Taking tiratricol along with stimulant drugs might cause serious problems including increased heart rate and high blood pressure. Avoid taking stimulant drugs along with tiratricol.

Some stimulant drugs include diethylpropion (Tenuate), epinephrine, phentermine (Ionamin), pseudoephedrine (Sudafed), and many others.

Thyroid hormone interacts with TIRATRICOL

Tiratricol works similarly to thyroid hormones. Taking tiratricol along with thyroid hormone pills might increase the chance of side effects from thyroid hormone.

Moderate Interaction Be cautious with this combination

Cholestyramine (Questran) interacts with TIRATRICOL

Cholestyramine (Questran) might decrease how much tiratricol the body absorbs. By decreasing how much tiratricol the body absorbs, cholestyramine (Questran) might decrease the effectiveness of tiratricol supplements. To avoid this interaction take tiratricol at least one hour before or four hours after taking cholestyramine.

Medications for diabetes (Antidiabetes drugs) interacts with TIRATRICOL

Large amounts of tiratricol can decrease blood sugar levels. Diabetes medications are also used to lower blood sugar. Taking tiratricol along with diabetes medications might cause your blood sugar to be too low. Monitor your blood sugar closely. The dose of your diabetes medication might need to be changed.

Some medications used for diabetes include glimepiride (Amaryl), glyburide (DiaBeta, Glynase PresTab, Micronase), insulin, pioglitazone (Actos), rosiglitazone (Avandia), chlorpropamide (Diabinese), glipizide (Glucotrol), tolbutamide (Orinase), and others.

Medications that slow blood clotting (Anticoagulant / Antiplatelet drugs) interacts with TIRATRICOL

Tiratricol might slow blood clotting. Taking tiratricol along with medications that also slow clotting might increase the chances of bruising and bleeding.

Some medications that slow blood clotting include aspirin, clopidogrel (Plavix), diclofenac (Voltaren, Cataflam, others), ibuprofen (Advil, Motrin, others), naproxen (Anaprox, Naprosyn, others), dalteparin (Fragmin), enoxaparin (Lovenox), heparin, warfarin (Coumadin), and others.

Source: WebMD
http://www.webmd.com/vitamins-supplements/ingredientmono-528-
TIRATRICOL.aspx?activeIngredientId=528&activeIngredientName=TIRATRICOL

YOHIMBINE

What is it?

Yohimbine is an extract of yohimbe bark, which is derived from the Corynanthe johimbe tree found in Africa.

What is it supposed to do?

Yohimbine is a metabolic stimulant like ephedrine and caffeine. As you may recall, I had mentioned that ephedrine is a beta–adrenergic agonist, which basically means it can stimulate something called a beta receptor found on various tissues in the body.

There are different sub-classes of beta receptors found on different tissues. It is these beta receptors that are affected by ephedrine, and that's how ephedrine ultimately causes fat loss, although it does have other systemic effects. Another class of receptors is called alpha receptors. Similar to beta receptors, there are several subtypes of alpha receptor found in different tissues.

Both the beta and the alpha receptors have a distinctive pattern of response to the catecholamines (i.e. adrenaline). Depending on which of these receptors you stimulate or block, different effects will be seen. Yohimbine is an alpha–2 adrenergic antagonist, which basically means it blocks the subtype 2 alpha receptors.

As alluded to in the ephedrine and caffeine section (EC), the topic of beta (and now alpha) adrenergic agonists and antagonists gets complicated rapidly.

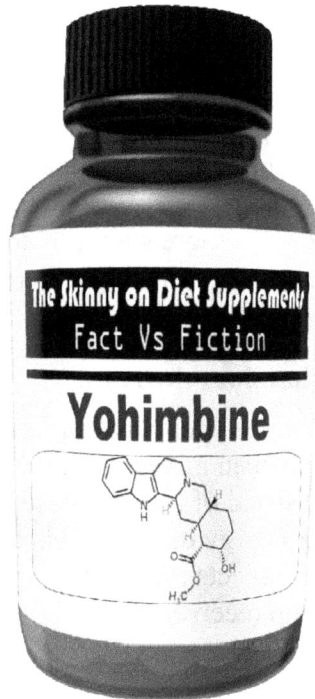

199

Lipolysis (the mobilization of stored body fat) can be initiated through stimulation of certain beta-adrenergic receptors or by inhibition of certain alpha adrenergic receptors.

Yohimbine is sold as a compound that can improve the effects of the EC based products and is often found combined with those ingredients. It's best known as a possible enhancer of libido in men and may have other medical uses. Some companies sell it as a testosterone booster and sports supplement.

Perhaps most interesting, the stubborn fat on women's thighs is more difficult to mobilize due to a high number and activity of these alpha-2 adrenergic receptors. Yohimbine may help to specifically reduce body fat in the more stubborn areas on women, which is most often the thighs and sides of the thighs known fondly as "saddle bags."

What does the research have to say?

Studies in humans that have looked at yohimbine as a weight loss agent have been mixed, with the majority finding no effects. One study with consisted of twenty obese female outpatients who were put on a 3 week, low energy diet (1,000 kcal/day) Using a double-blind study protocol, ten subjects received 5 mg yohimbine 4 times a day while the other group received a placebo for three weeks, in addition to a low calorie diet.

The study found the yohimbine "significantly increased weight loss" in the group getting the supplement. However, several other studies utilizing larger groups of both men and women, found no effects on weight loss with yohimbine supplements.

Several animal studies have found yohimbine has an anorectic (appetite suppressive) quality and dogs fed yohimbine ate less food and lost weight.

One study that tried to use yohimbine as a topical "thigh cream" but found no effects on fat loss in the thighs or systemically (Interestingly, other ingredients did appear to work for spot reduction, but this is not an book about fat loss creams, so I will end the discussion of topical creams here).

200

Of particular importance and concern to the dieter using EC based products, is that it was found that yohimbine added to EC impaired cardiac performance and reduced the ejection fraction of the heart.

A similar group in the study getting only EC found no such effects on the vascular system and heart.

Theoretically, yohimbine should assist in weight loss when combined with EC, but there is little proof or research to show it. Studies on yohimbine alone for weight loss have been mixed or unimpressive.

Some in-vitro (test tube) studies suggest yohimbine can reduce fat synthesis and have other effects that should increase fat oxidation (fat "burning").

Studies using yohimbine to boost male libido have been promising, and there is a prescription strength product doctors can prescribe for that use. Yohimbine appears to increase blood flow to the penis while decreasing blood flow out, thus making an erection easier and "better." Some cultures consider yohimbe bark to be a real aphrodisiac.

As indicated above, yohimbine works through non-sex hormone pathways and studies have found it does not increase testosterone.

Other studies have shown yohimbine can reduce platelet aggregation, thus potentially lowering the risk of heart attacks and strokes (similar to aspirin's effects on the blood but by another mechanism). Other studies have found yohimbine to be useful in the treatment of congestive heart failure.

What does the real world say for weight loss?

People who have mixed yohimbine with EC based products generally feel it has an additive effect for weight loss. Very few people take yohimbine alone for weight loss, so there is little feedback on that score.

Will Brink's Recommendation

On paper and in theory, yohimbine should be helpful for weight loss, especially when mixed with EC products. However, one plus one rarely makes two in the human body. It often makes three, and sometimes one and a half, but rarely two.

Also, as mentioned in the section on ephedrine and caffeine, there are only so many stimulants you can put in the system, and the above study would seem to suggest that EC and yohimbine combined may be potentially problematic to the heart and vascular system of some people. It makes sense that certain stimulants just don't combine well while others work fine without serious side effects.

My advice to people who want to mix yohimbine and other natural stimulants (i.e. ephedrine, caffeine, etc.) would be to reduce the dose of the other products to half their normal recommended dose and add in the yohimbine cautiously. Though the positive effects on weight loss of the EC based products may be enhanced by the use of yohimbine, one of the possible side effects could be additive.

My advice for yohimbine is going to be similar for that of ephedrine, or any stimulant for that matter. People who don't tolerate stimulants well, people with pre-existing medical conditions such as heart disease or heart irregularities, high blood pressure, or prostate disease and pregnant women, or people taking MAO inhibitors are advised to avoid such products or to use caution and a little common sense.

One important issue to remember is that studies looking at weight loss have used pure yohimbine, not the yohimbe bark that is found in health food stores. Yohimbe supplements are notorious for containing little if any actual yohimbine. Even good quality yohimbe supplements are approximately 3-4% actual yohimbine.

This means, if the product actually contains 4% active yohimbine, it will take 300 mg of ground bark to get just 12 mg of yohimbine.

Most studies have used doses ranging from 10 mg per day in two doses (i.e. 2 x 5 mg) up to 40 mg per day in divided doses. I would consider 40 mg far too high a dose for long term safety. If combined with EC-based products, 10 mg–20 mg/day of yohimbine in divided doses would be the upper limit.

However, the response to such products is very individual. Lower doses of yohimbine should be attempted to see if any undesirable side effects occur. Translated, some people can drink a pot of coffee at night and go to sleep while others can't tolerate a single cup of coffee at any time.

At reasonable doses in healthy people, yohimbine appears quite safe. However, mixed with other products or taken by people with pre-existing medical issues, the margin of safety is likely to drop. This is something to keep in mind if you're considering mixing various products together.

Possible Drug Interactions to be aware of

Major Interaction Do not take this combination

Medications for depression (MAOIs) interacts with YOHIMBE

Yohimbe contains a chemical that affects the body. This chemical is called yohimbine. Yohimbine might affect the body in some of the same ways as some medications for depression called MAOIs. Taking yohimbe along with MAOIs might increase the effects and side effects of yohimbe and MAOIs.

Some of these medications used for depression include phenelzine (Nardil), tranylcypromine (Parnate), and others.

Moderate Interaction Be cautious with this combination

Clonidine (Catapres) interacts with YOHIMBE

Clonidine (Catapres) is used to decrease blood pressure. Yohimbe might increase blood pressure. Taking yohimbe along with clonidine (Catapres) might decrease the effectiveness of clonidine (Catapres).

Guanabenz (Wytensin) interacts with YOHIMBE

Yohimbe contains a chemical called yohimbine. Yohimbine can decrease the effectiveness of guanabenz (Wytensin).

Medications for depression (Tricyclic antidepressants) interacts with YOHIMBE

Yohimbe can affect the heart. Some medications used for depression called tricyclic antidepressants can also affect the heart. Taking yohimbe along with these medications used for depression might cause heart problems. Don't take yohimbe if you are taking these medications for depression.

Some of these tricyclic antidepressants medications used for depression include amitriptyline (Elavil), imipramine (Tofranil), and others.

Medications for high blood pressure (Antihypertensive drugs) interacts with YOHIMBE

Yohimbe seems to increase blood pressure. Taking yohimbe along with some medications for high blood pressure might decrease the effectiveness of medications for high blood pressure.

Some medications for high blood pressure include captopril (Capoten), enalapril (Vasotec), losartan (Cozaar), valsartan (Diovan), diltiazem (Cardizem), amlodipine (Norvasc), hydrochlorothiazide (HydroDiuril), furosemide (Lasix), and many others.

Naloxone (Narcan) interacts with YOHIMBE

Yohimbe contains a chemical that can affect the brain. This chemical is called yohimbine. Naloxone (Narcan) also affects the brain. Taking naloxone (Narcan) along with yohimbine might increase the chance of side effects such as anxiety, nervousness, trembling, and hot flashes.

Phenothiazines interacts with YOHIMBE

Yohimbe contains a chemical called yohimbine. Some medications called phenothiazines have some similar effects to yohimbine. Taking yohimbe along with phenothiazines might increase the effects and side effects of yohimbine.

   Some phenothiazines include chlorpromazine (Thorazine), fluphenazine (Prolixin), trifluoperazine (Stelazine), thioridazine (Mellaril), and others.

Stimulant drugs interacts with YOHIMBE

Stimulant drugs speed up the nervous system. By speeding up the nervous system, stimulant medications can make you feel jittery and speed up your heartbeat. Yohimbe might also speed up the nervous system. Taking yohimbe along with stimulant drugs might cause serious problems including increased heart rate and high blood pressure. Avoid taking stimulant drugs along with yohimbe.

Some stimulant drugs include diethylpropion (Tenuate), epinephrine, phentermine (Ionamin), pseudoephedrine (Sudafed), and many others.

Source: http://www.webmd.com/vitamins-supplements/ingredientmono-759-YOHIMBE.aspx?activeIngredientId=759&activeIngredientName=YOHIMBE

SUPPLEMENT SCORECARD

Now that you've read the reviews, you're ready to go shopping, right?

I can hear it now: "Will, you've got to be kidding me! There are over 150 pages of supplement information! How am I supposed to remember all that?"

The good news is: you don't have to. That's what this "Supplement Scorecard" is for— so you can see at a glance what is recommended, what might be worth a try, and what isn't worth the money. I've also listed the currently recommended amounts, so you can see if the supplement you're considering is providing useful ingredients and useful doses.

Remember, this scorecard only takes into account a supplement's potential effects on weight loss, and not other potential uses for improving health or performance.

Readers using this scorecard should not overlook a supplement's uses for other things, or potential side effects which are outlined in the full description of each supplement in the book.

Supplements/nutrients worth using

EC-based formulas

Recommended Dose: 200 mg caffeine/20 mg ephedrine, 3 times/day before meals or exercise.* Cycle 8-14 weeks on/2-6 weeks off. **See warnings for who should not use EC based products**

Fish Oil, Udo's Choice, Flax oil

Recommended Dose:
Fish oil: 6-10 g/day.
Udo's Choice: 1 tbsp. per 50 lbs. bodyweight.
Flax: 1 tbsp. per 75 lbs. bodyweight.

Green Tea extracts

Use an amount equivalent to 90 mg EGCG 3 times/day.

Tyrosine

Recommended Dose: Use 500-1000 mg, 2-3 times/day, 30-40 minutes before meals on an empty stomach.

Whey Protein:

Recommended Dose: Use as needed/desired for additional protein.

206

Could be worth a try but needs more research

CLA
Recommended Dose: least 3 g/day (4-6 g/day preferred).

7-Keto DHEA
Recommended Dose: Take 100-200 mg/day in divided doses.

Forskolin
Recommended Dose: Use 250 mg of 10% extract (25 mg) twice/day

GMP
Recommended Dose: 3 scoops whey/day, taken 30-40 minutes prior to meals. Also see whey side bar.

Glucomannan
Recommended Dose: 3 grams before meals; take w/10 oz. of water

5–HTP
Recommended Dose: Take 200-300 mg before meals, 3 times per day.

Guggul/Phosphate
Recommended Dose: 6 capsules/day with meals (i.e., 2 capsules taken 3 times/day).

Peptide FM
Recommended Dose: Take 1-4 g/day.

Synephrine

Recommended Dose: 4-20 mg/day (200-600 mg Citrus aurantium extract standardized to 3-6% synephrine).

Medium Chain Triglycerides (MCTs)

Recommended Dose: up to 3tbs per day or as tolerated.

Yohimbine

Recommended Dose: Use 10-20 mg/day in divided doses.

Probably not worth spending money on (for weight loss)

Carnitine	Insulin Potentiators
Cayenne (capsaicin)	Lipotropics
Acetyl-L-Carnitine	Octopamine
Chromium	Orlistat
Chitosan	Phaseolus vulgaris extract
Co-enzyme Q10	Phosphatidylserine
DHEA	Piperine
Digestive enzymes	Pyruvate
Evodiamine/evodia	Salvia sclarea
Hoodia	Tetradecylthioacetic acid
GH releasing nutrients	Thyromimetics
HCA	Sesamin

USING THE SUPPLEMENT SCORECARD

To illustrate how the Scorecard can be used to evaluate a supplement, we'll apply the information to a commercial product that I'll call *"Fat Burner Extreme"* for the purposes of this discussion.

Let's take a look at the ingredients and dosage instructions:

Supplement Facts:

Serving Size: 2 Capsules
Servings Per Container: 60

       Amount Per Serving:
ForsLean® Coleus Forskohlii Extract: 62.5 mg
 [standardized for 40% forskohlin (25 mg)]
Guarana Extract: 228 mg
 [standardized for 22% alkaloids as caffeine (50 mg)]
Gymnema Sylvestre Extract: 100 mg
 [standardized for 25% gymnemic acids (25 mg)]
Citrus Aurantium Extract: 94 mg
 [standardized for 8% synephrine (7.5 mg)]
Green Tea Extract: 60 mg
 [standardized for 50% polyphenols extract (30 mg)]
USP Caffeine: 50 mg
Calcium Phosphate: 764 mg
Bioperine: 2.5mg

Other Ingredients:
Silica Dioxide, Magnesium Stearate and Gelatin(capsule).

Directions: As a dietary supplement, take 2 capsules twice daily with meals.

The first ingredient is *ForsLean®*, which supplies 25 mg (62.5 mg of a 40% extract) forskolin in each two capsule serving. Forskolin is rated "could be worth a try." Since the supplement instructions state: "take 2 capsules twice daily" this matches the recommended dose in the Supplement Scoreboard: 25 mg twice/day.

Guarana extract is next: guarana is a source of caffeine, and the extract provides 50 mg of it. If you look down the list, you'll also see that another 50 mg of "USP Caffeine" is included—which brings the total dose of caffeine to 100 mg. This is the caffeine equivalent to about half a cup of coffee—not a huge amount.

Gymnema sylvestre extract is the third ingredient: if you recall from the review section, this is an insulin potentiator. It's on the "probably not worth spending money on" list, as there's no proof it will help with fat loss—although it might help control blood sugar levels.

Citrus aurantium extract is next on the list: 94 mg supplies 7.5 mg of synephrine. Synephrine is also on the "could be worth a try" list, and a range of 4–20 mg/day is suggested. The total daily dose provided by *"Fat Burner Extreme"* is 15 mg: which is at the higher end of the recommended range.

Green tea extract is one of the "supplements/nutrients worth using", but *"Fat Burner Extreme"* only supplies 30 mg. of total polyphenols, and the extract is not standardized for EGCG. The recommended amount of EGCG alone is 90 mg, taken 3 times/day, so this ingredient is definitely underdosed!

Calcium phosphate is not on our supplement list, nor does it need to be – most people know what it is and what it's good for. Calcium is a useful nutrient that many people don't get enough of. Calcium from dairy products can enhance fat loss, but, calcium supplements are less effective.

So while calcium is a useful nutrient from a health perspective, there's little to be gained (or lost) by including it.

The final ingredient is *Bioperine* which is the name of a commercial piperine extract. It's also on the "probably not worth spending money on" list.

210

So what can we conclude about *"Fat Burner Extreme"?*

We have 2 ingredients that "could be worth a try," a modest amount of caffeine, several questionable nutrients and one nutrient that's "worth using" but is significantly under dosed, so based on what you now know from this book, *"Fat Burner Extreme"* doesn't look very impressive at all.

In my opinion, any additional fat loss beyond what you'd get from diet and exercise alone is likely to be limited. I'd save my money and look for something else.

See how this works? With a little practice, you'll be an expert—and save yourself a lot of money in the process.

FOR MORE INFORMATION

For more information, check out the BrinkZone.com

There you will find free reports, additional articles, videos, and other resources that will help you save money, and stop the wasted time on potentially worthless supplements!

Also see the other links below to get additional information.

INFORMATION ON SUPPLEMENTS

http://www.creatine-report.com

http://www.BrinkZone.com

STUDIES AND OTHER SCIENTIFIC DATA

http://www.ncbi.nlm.nih.gov/pubmed/

INDEX

D

E

F

www.ingramcontent.com/pod-product-compliance
Lightning Source LLC
Chambersburg PA
CBHW070910270326
41927CB00011B/2517